Books and other resources may be ordered through book sellers or by contacting:
www.sheilagunlock.com
1-417-986-1998

MORE BOOKS BY SHEILA GUNLOCK
Growing up Great with Groovy Granny - 2011
Mt See-More Adventure– 2023
Sea Odyssey Puppet Script – 2023
Missouri Maggie Puppet Script – 2024

Author – Sheila Gunlock
Illustrator – Shea Dalton Piercy

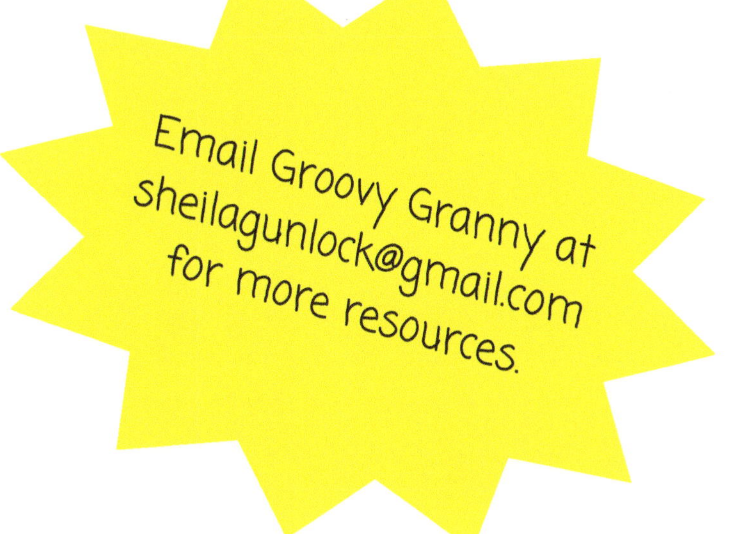

This book is dedicated to
all of our little superheroes
fighting the fight of the Grub Bugs!
And to all of us who fuel their mission
sending them into their future in good health!
We can create a better world when we
share our wisdom, knowledge and
most importantly, our love.

Groovy Granny

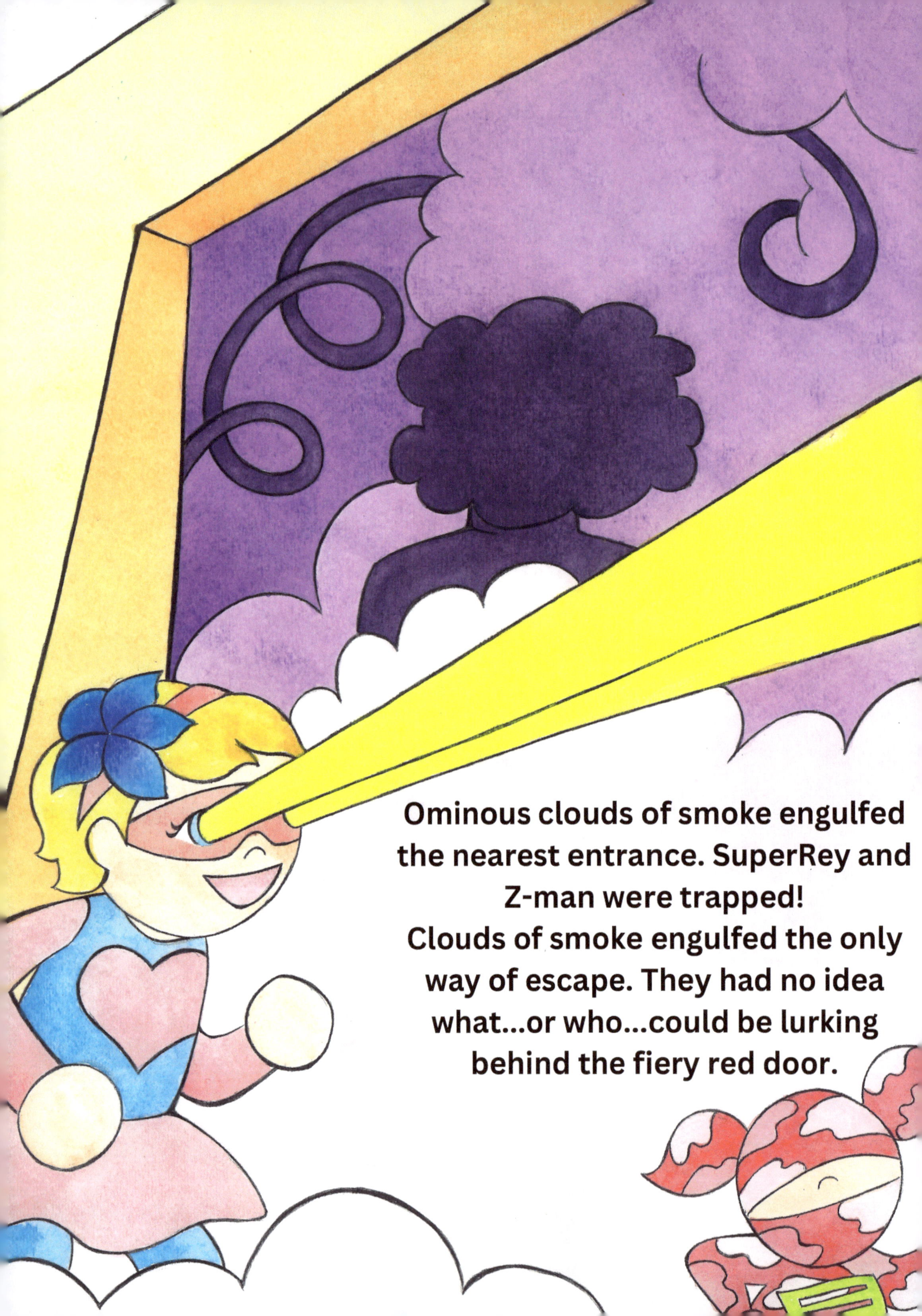

Ominous clouds of smoke engulfed the nearest entrance. SuperRey and Z-man were trapped!
Clouds of smoke engulfed the only way of escape. They had no idea what...or who...could be lurking behind the fiery red door.

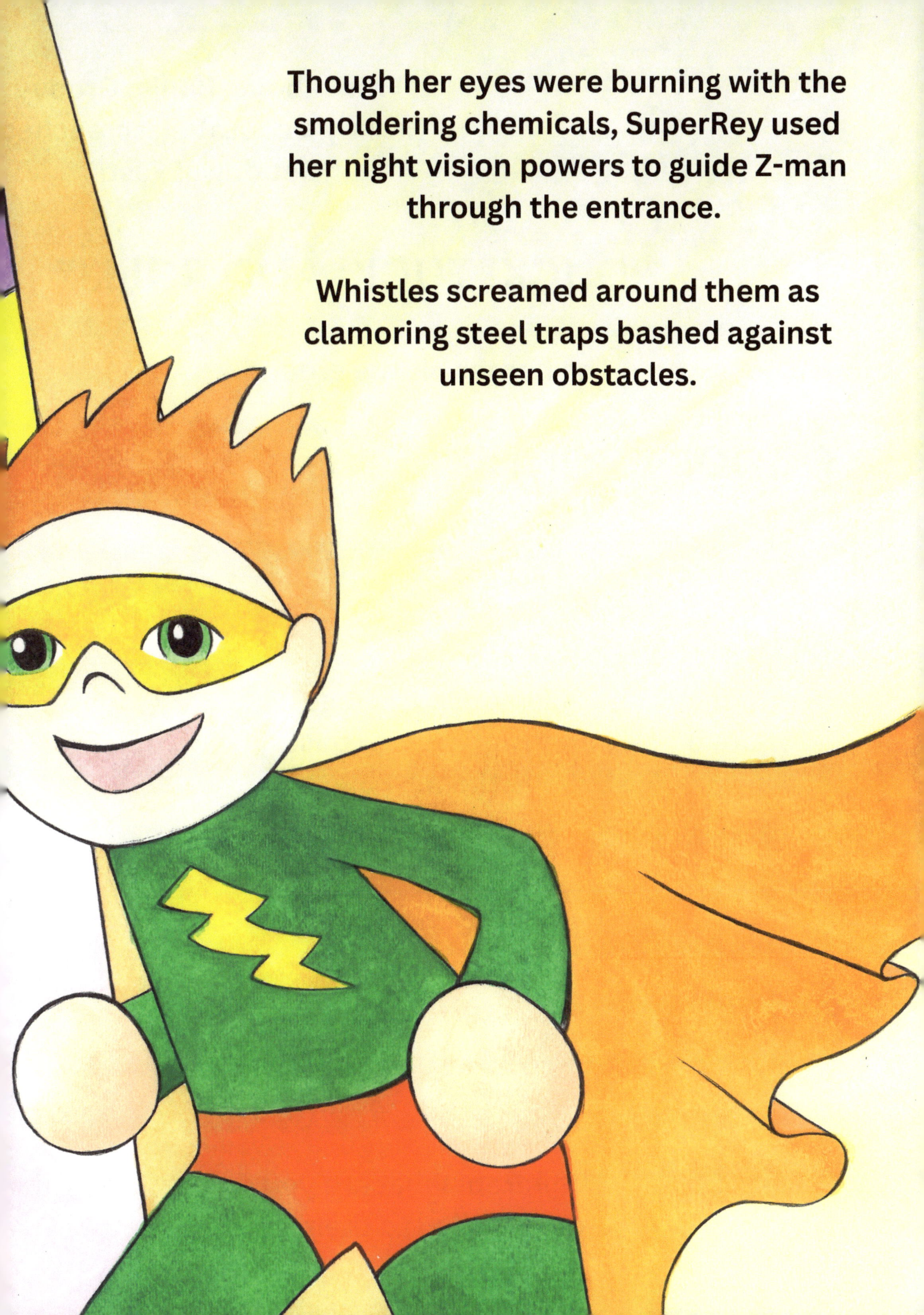

Though her eyes were burning with the smoldering chemicals, SuperRey used her night vision powers to guide Z-man through the entrance.

Whistles screamed around them as clamoring steel traps bashed against unseen obstacles.

From above, Banjo, Groovy Granny's cockatiel, screeched "Get down! Fast!"

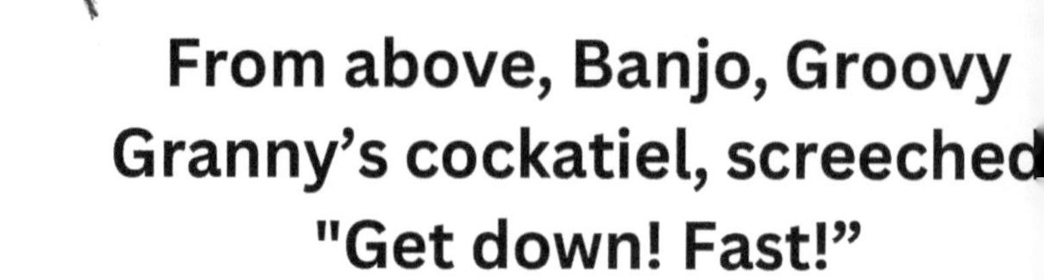

"DUCK! TUCK! AND ROLL!"

The heroes hit the ground.

OOOOF!! OOHH!!

In that same split second, a huge white billowy contraption flew past, just above them.

"Children! What are you doing?" a familiar voice called to them in the distance.

"Groovy Granny! It's us, Reyah Hope and Zacker-Doodle. Where are you?" shouted Reyah above the smoke and bangs.

"Children, stay where you are."

WHIRRRRRR!!

ZZZZRRRROOOOOOOMMMMMMM. . .

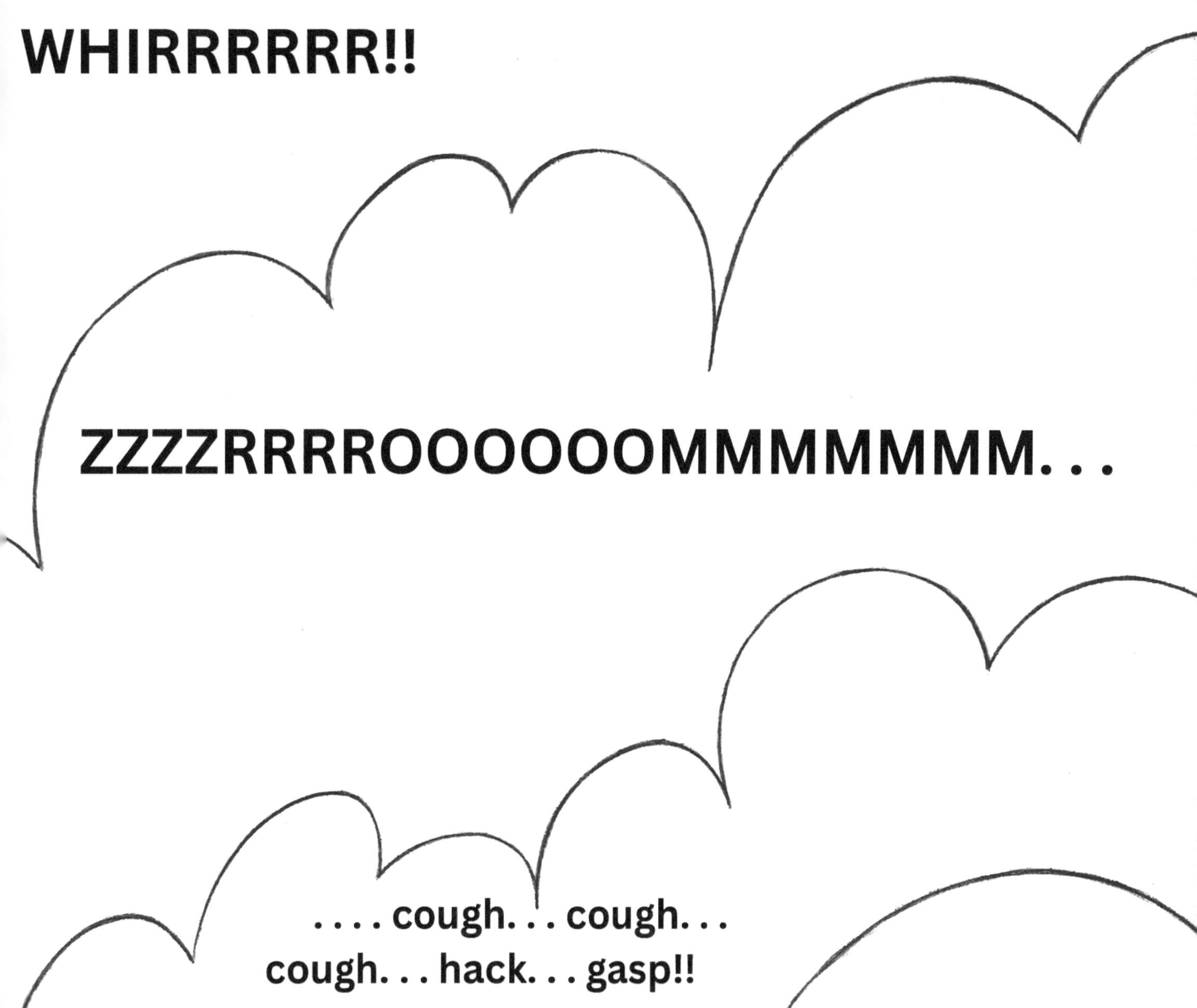

. . . . cough. . . cough. . . cough. . . hack. . . gasp!!

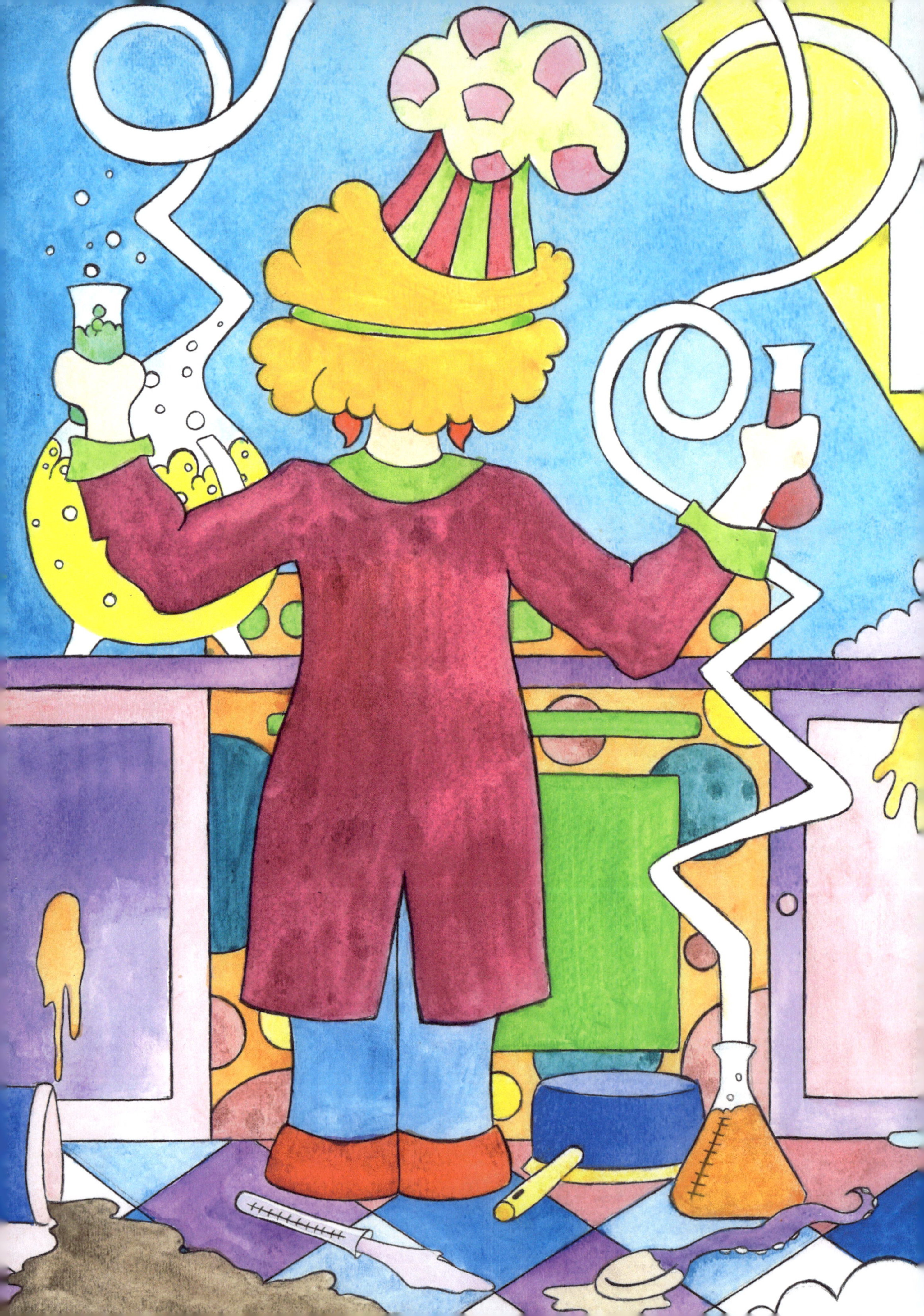

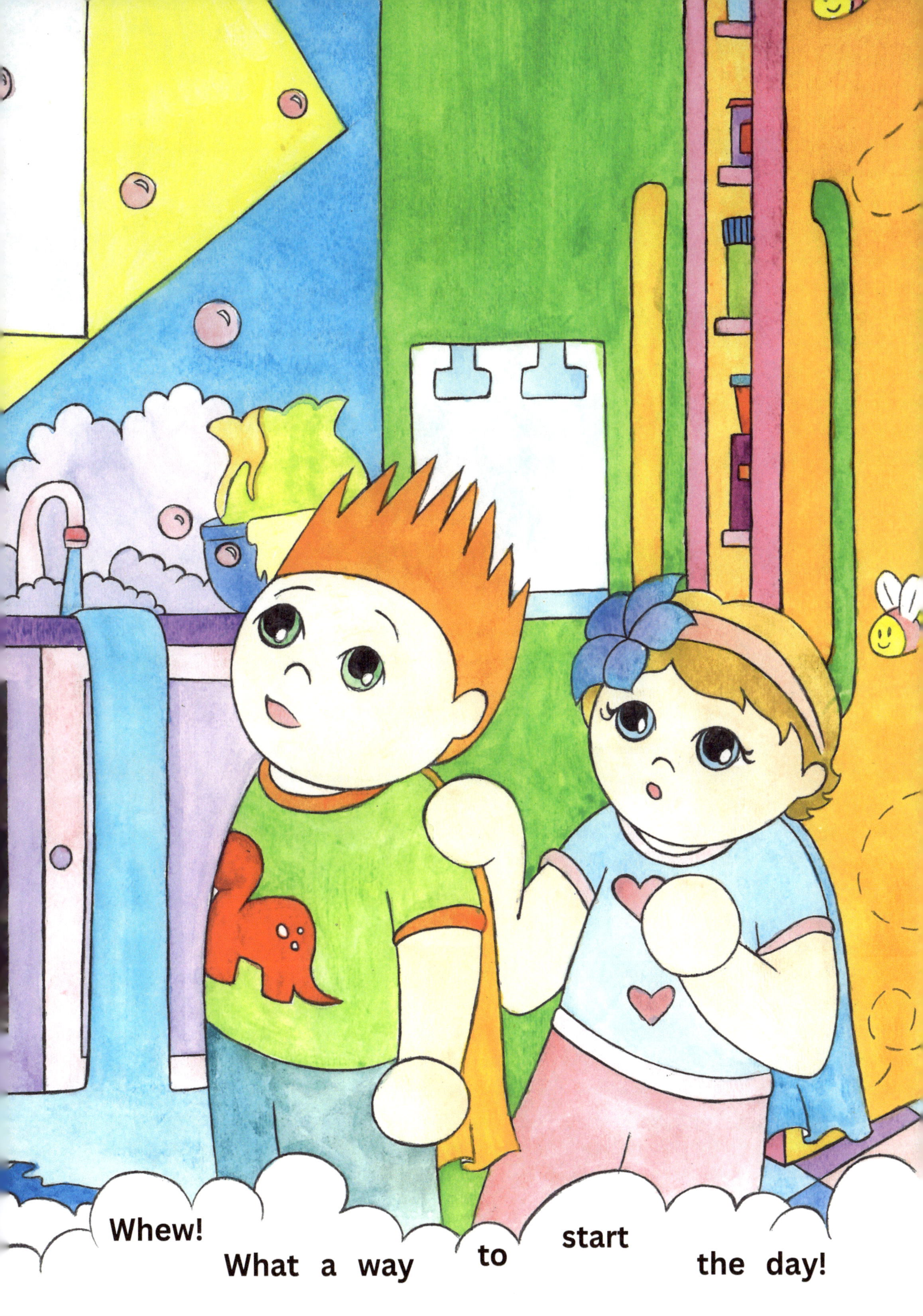
Whew!
What a way to start the day!

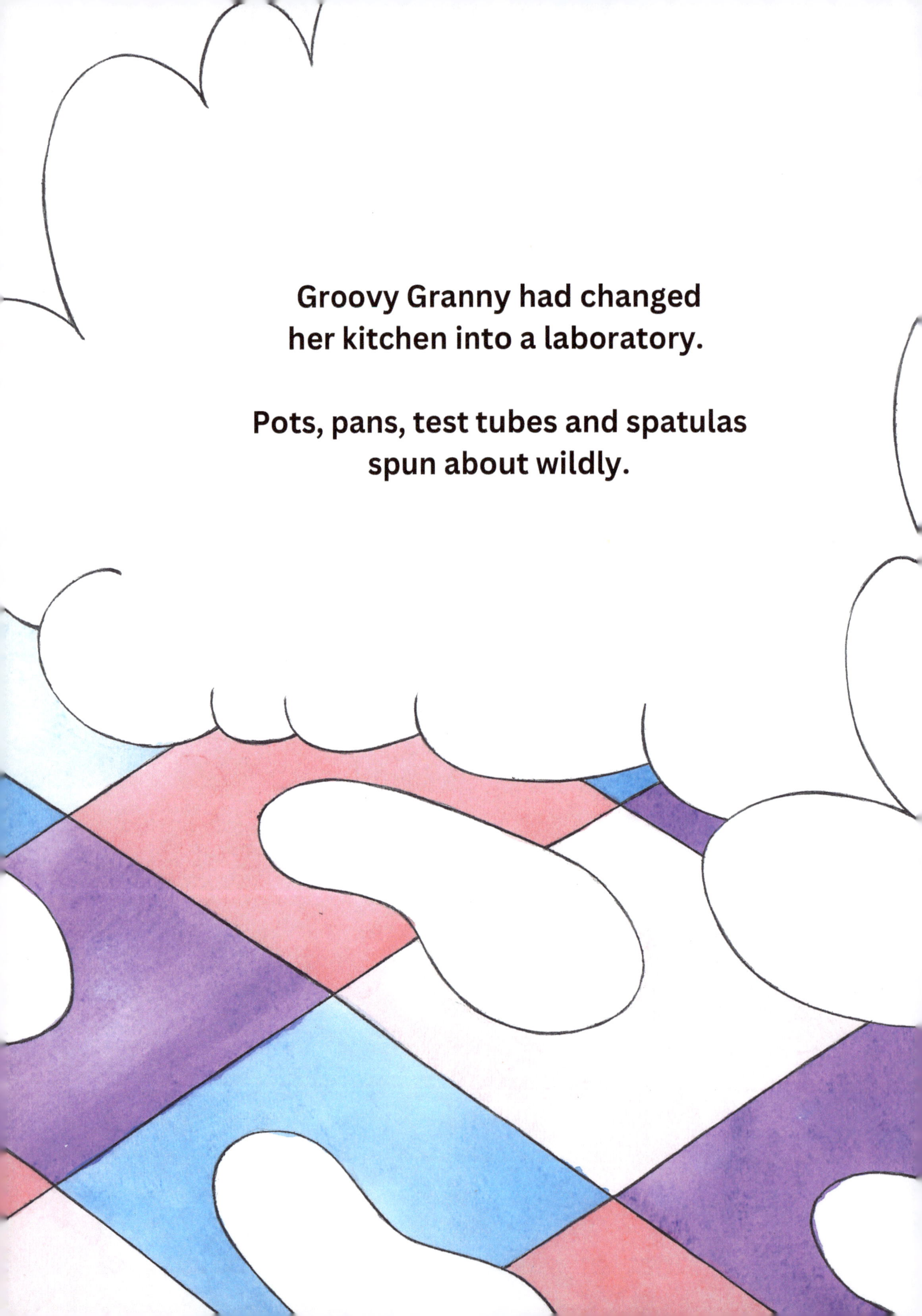

Groovy Granny had changed
her kitchen into a laboratory.

Pots, pans, test tubes and spatulas
spun about wildly.

"Is everything alright? Banjo? Reyah Hope?
Zacker-Doodle? Lola?"

Zacker-Doodle checked out the mess on the
floor as he straightened out his new Z-man cape.
"Yep, they sure are.
What's all the smoke for?"

But before Groovy Granny could answer. . .

"Ohhhh myyy!"
cried Lola

"Groovy Granny, what a mess!"
proclaimed Reyah.

They had never seen Groovy Granny's kitchen
look this dirty. . .
EVER!

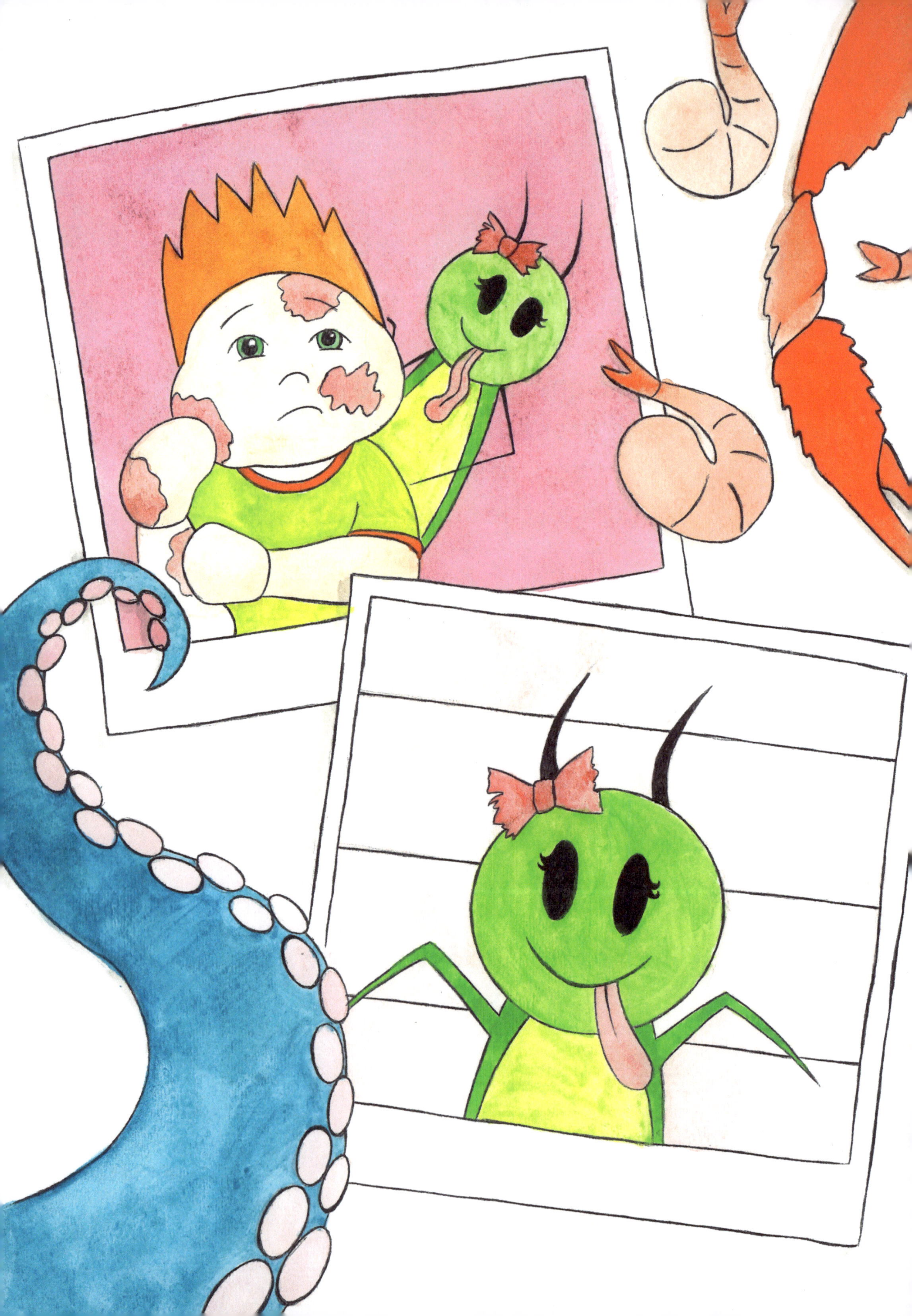

"I have just discovered the secret 'itchy' formula that Bea Hive uses to make people's skin break out in hives and itch like crazy," answered Groovy Granny.

"Hives? " Zacker-Doodle asked. He suddenly realized the smoke was just flour. He made footprints in the white flour on the kitchen floor.

"Yes," said Granny. "Hives are when you get big, red bumps on your skin."

Zacker-Doodle scratched his arm, "Yeah, then we itch and wiggle and wiggle and itch!"

"Well children, it's a good thing you came over today ready to be HEROES!" Groovy Granny explained what had happened this morning. "Do my heroes remember the notorious Grub Bug Gang that we fought a couple of years ago?"

"I do! The Choker wouldn't let me breathe," remembered Reyah.

Reyah moved closer to Groovy Granny. Just the thought of it made her shudder. "I never want to feel that way again! The Choker made my throat get super tight. My mouth felt funny and tingly. My heart was beating really fast. And my head hurt. I didn't know peanuts could do that to some people. I'm glad you knew what to do, Groovy Granny."

"We learned what the Grub Bugs could do to some people. But Grub Bugs can't hurt everyone," said Groovy Granny.

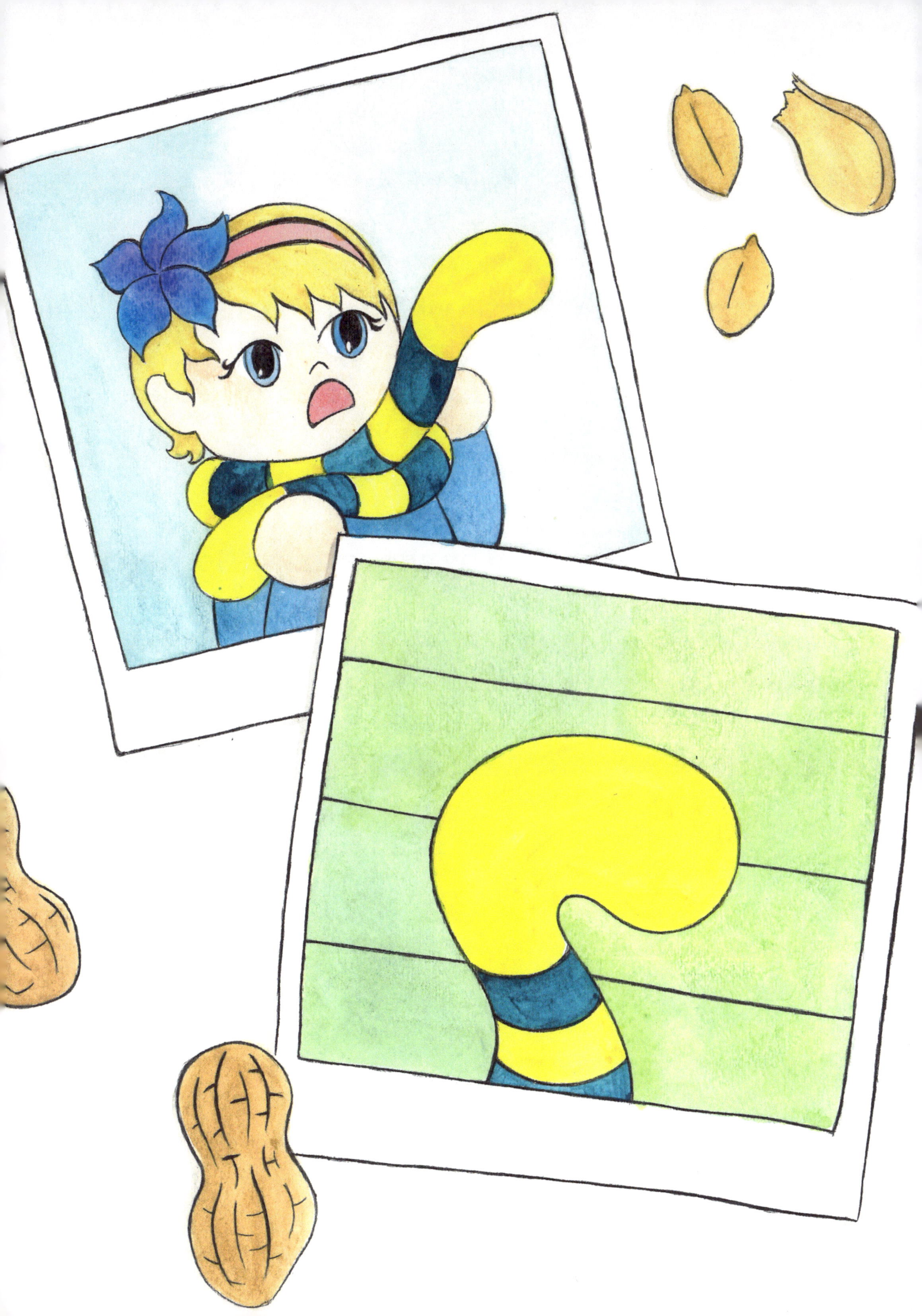

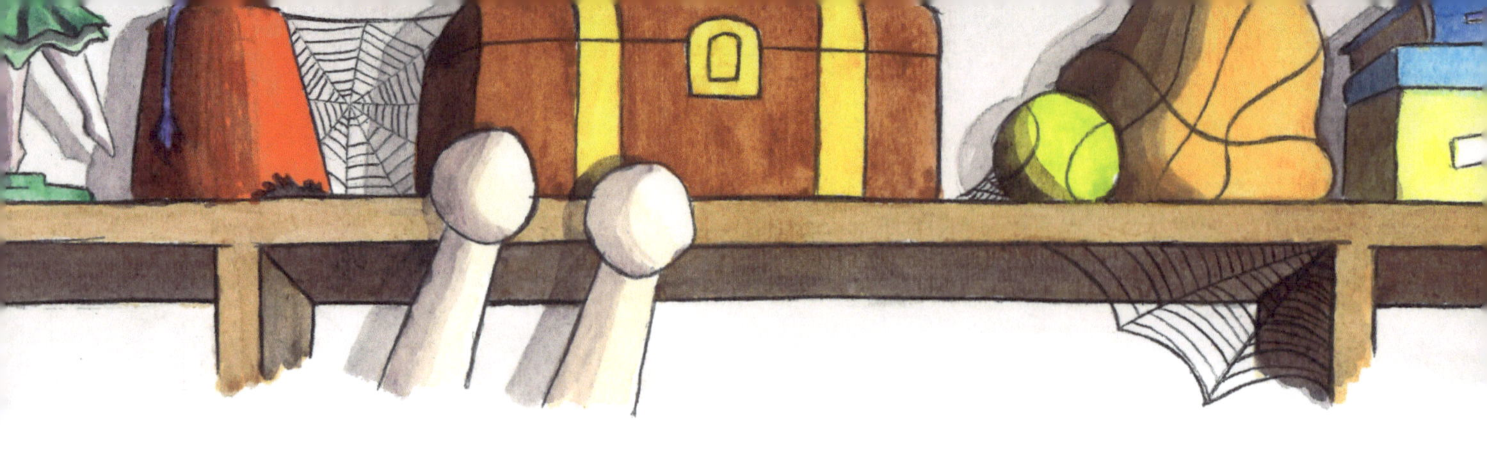

With a swift spin, Z-man whipped his cape around and in his best hero voice declared, "Together, we foiled those evil villains. Haaahaaa! We trapped those Grub Bugs! And put them away where they couldn't hurt anyone anymore. Right?"

Banjo swooped by all in a tizzy. "No, No, No!"

Banjo screeched. "Lola found them! Oh dear, oh dear! She thought I hid her camo baseball cap up there. The box looked like a treasure chest. Oh dear, oh dear! Nothing stops Lola when she is after her hat.
Oh dear, oh dear!
CRRAAAASSSSHH!! BANGGGGG!!
SCREEEEEAAAMMMMM!!
It's awful!"

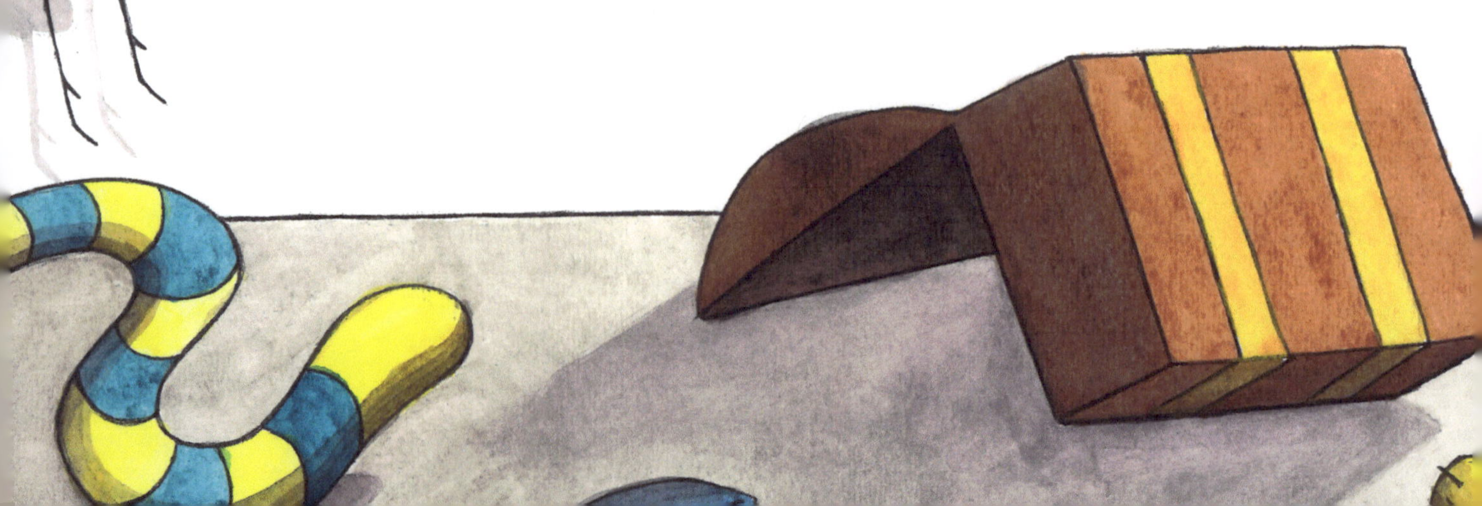

"I heard a terrible commotion," Groovy Granny said.
"I ran down the cellar stairs to find a dazed Lola
and a screaming Banjo.
Even worse, I found the empty lock box
where the Grub Bugs had been trapped!
I know the Grub Bugs will attack again.
We must do something before it's too late!"

"Don't worry Groovy Granny, they can't get to Lola.
We will get her a hero cape
and she will be even stronger!"
Zacker-Doodle said with great determination.

"You're right. There's not much that can stop
Lola, but those Grub Bugs can," explained Groovy
Granny. "The Grub Bugs find a weakness in a
person's body to make us sick,
weak, or even worse."

"If Lola eats bananas, that Itchy Bug wiggles in there
and makes her tongue and throat itchy.
Have you ever tried to scratch your tongue without
using your fingers? Or scratching your throat
on the INSIDE?
Sometimes Lola makes a gurgling sound
to scratch the Itchy places in her throat.
If it's really bad, she makes a growly, screechy
sound," Groovy Granny explained.
"That's when the Itchy Bug attacks. No one has ever
seen the Itchy Bug, but from all the clues we have,
I imagine it looks like a caterpillar."

". . . then with its prickly tickly spines, curling and
swirling around until it gets comfortable,
its spines begin to quiver and that makes Lola itchy.
And this is no slow caterpillar. It all happens
lightning fast!" said Groovy Granny.

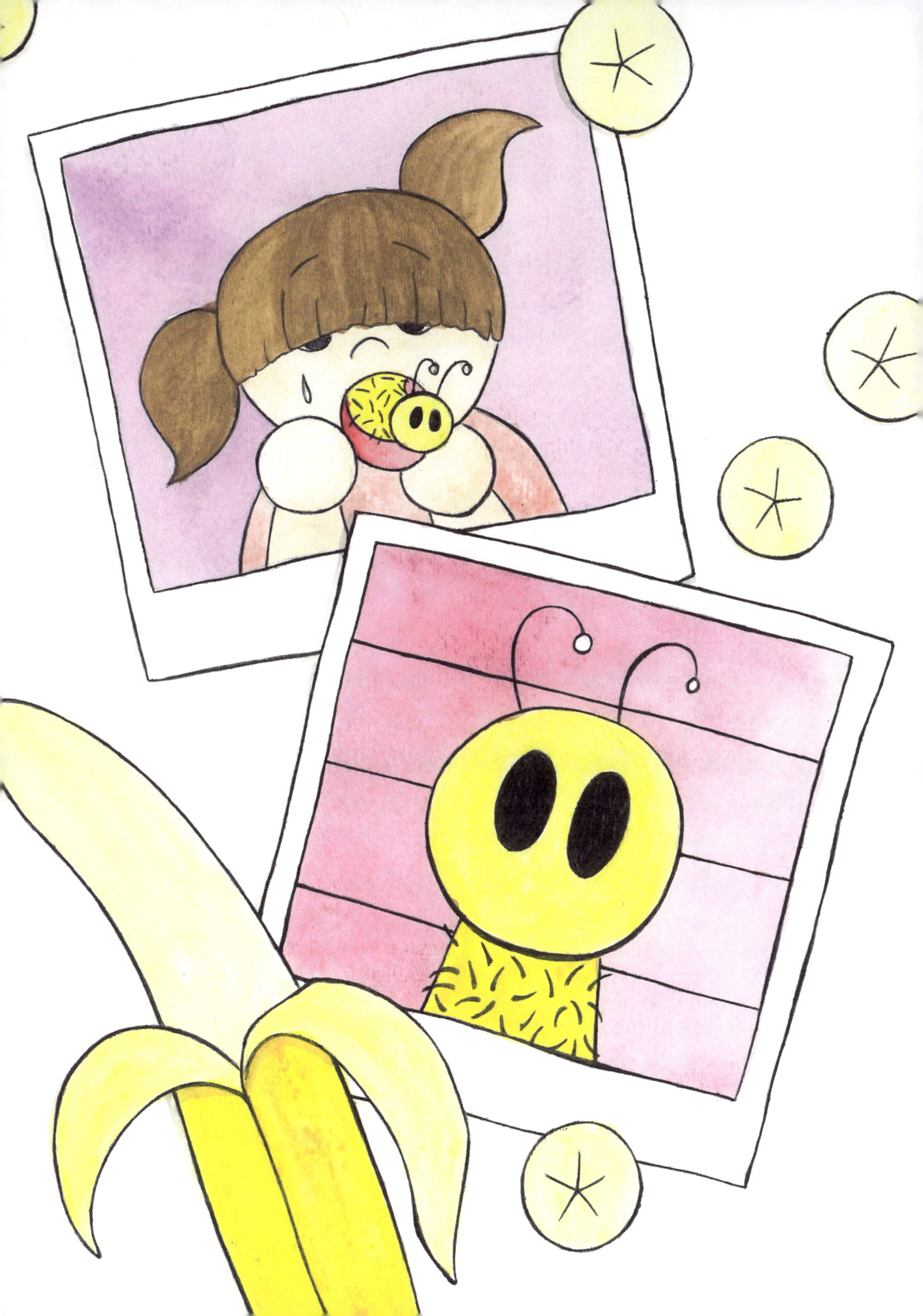

"Just give me the chance! Face to face!" Z-man paused, "Oh... does the Itchy Bug have a face?" asked Zacker-Doodle. "With my superpowers, I can go in circles, like a tornado. All that twisting will tie that bug in a knot so he can't make anyone itchy."

"But Zacker, if that bug can get in Lola's throat, we are too big to fight it.
We just need to step on it!" reasoned Reyah.

Determined, Zacker-Doodle replied, "I'm sure he can make himself big OR little to get where he wants to go so he can make people itchy. When he came out and was big again, I would be there to tie him up!"

"Well, if you don't stop spinning right now, we won't be able to find Banjo in all that white flour fog," laughed Groovy Granny.

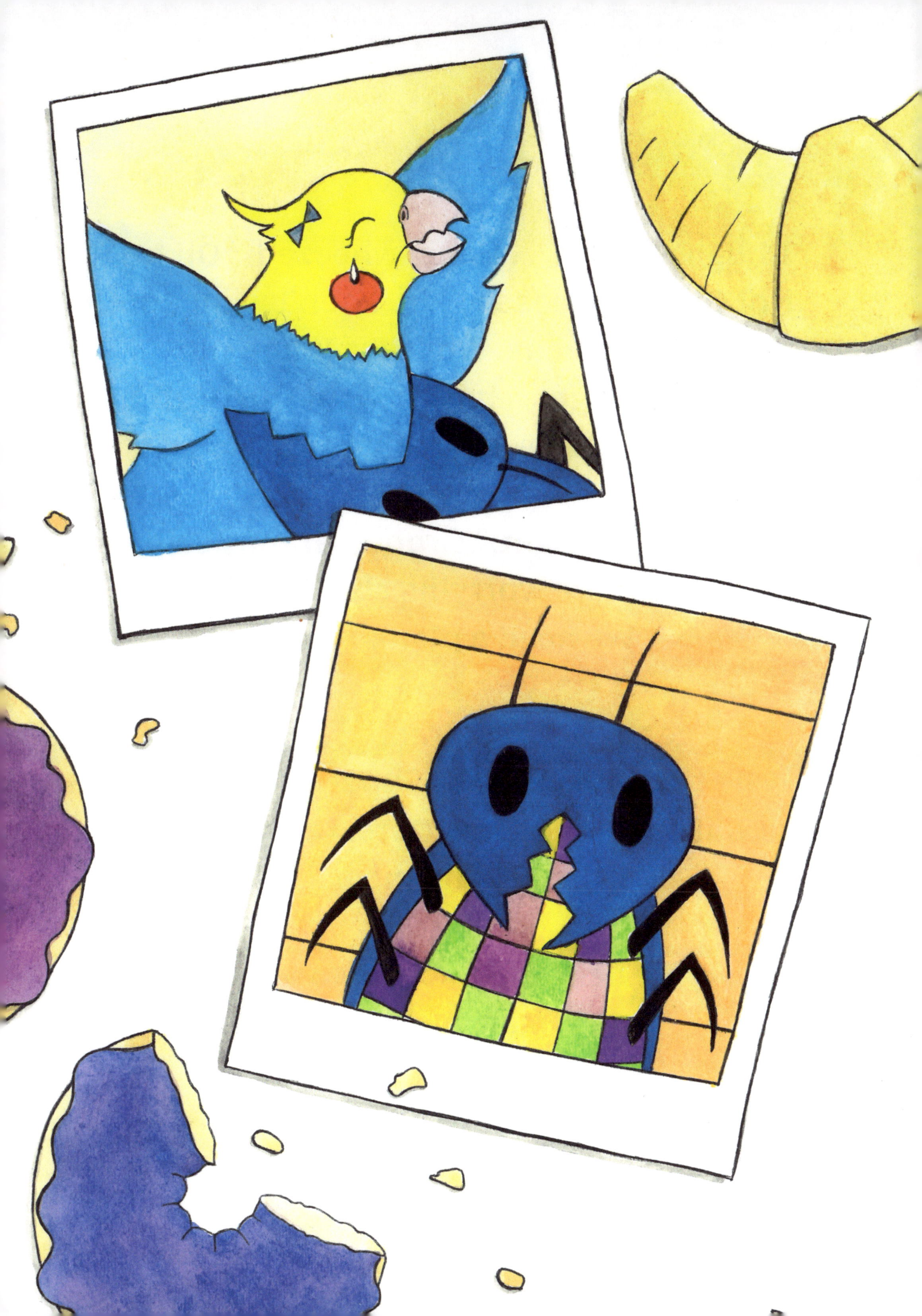

Cough... cough. . . Banjo wheezed, "Oh No! Oh No! Gutter is loose again. I don't want another stomachache. While we figure out. . . cough. . . cough. . . how to fight the Grub Bugs, they know exactly what to do to US!"

"Banjo's right," Groovy Granny said.
"No more worrying about the past.
We need a plan of attack!"

"I got it, Groovy Granny!" Lola squealed as she transformed into Super Lola Ninja Girl. "I will catch those cwitters. I am not afwaid of them no mowa!"

"Me neither!" exclaimed SuperRey
and Z-man at the same time.

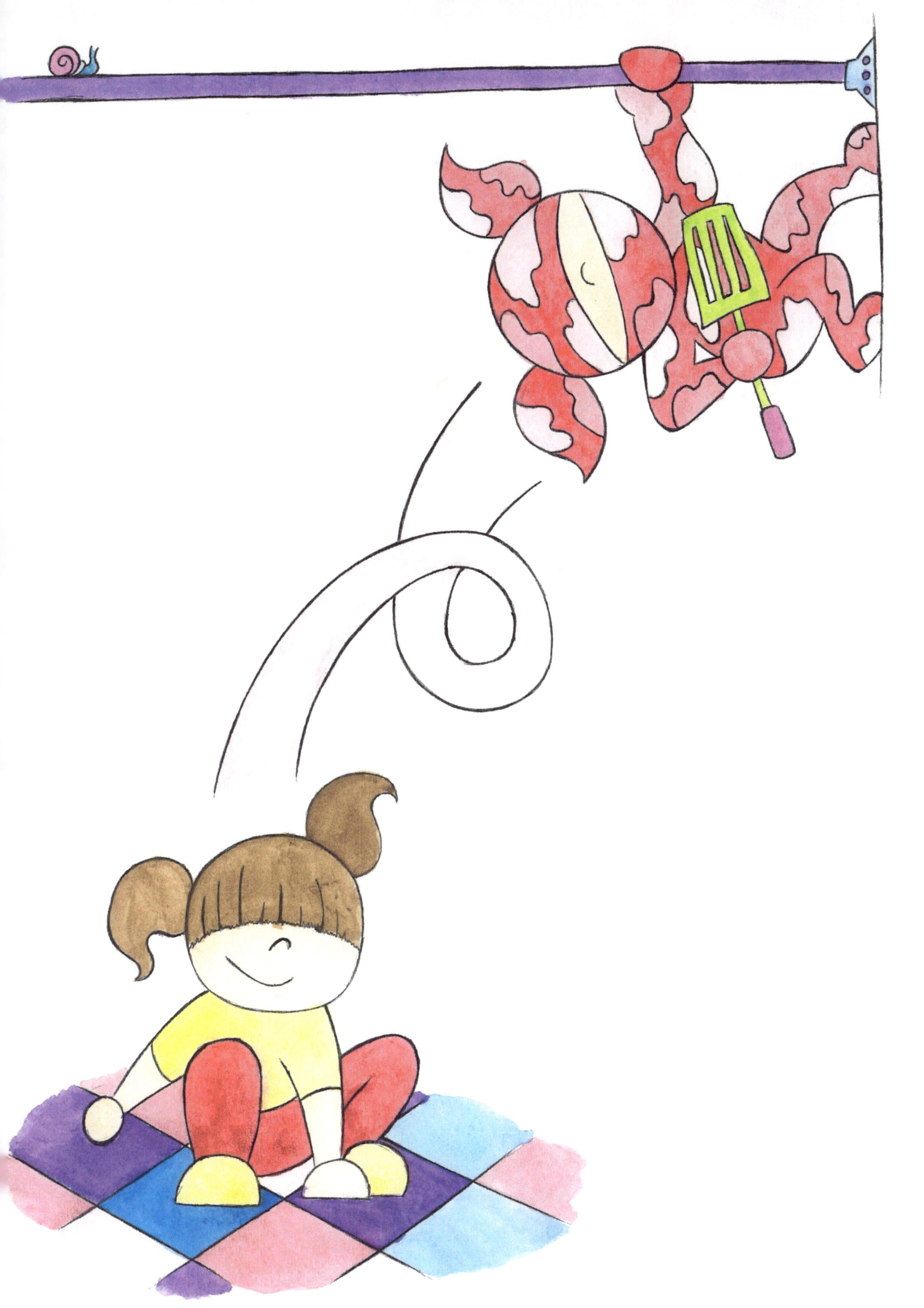

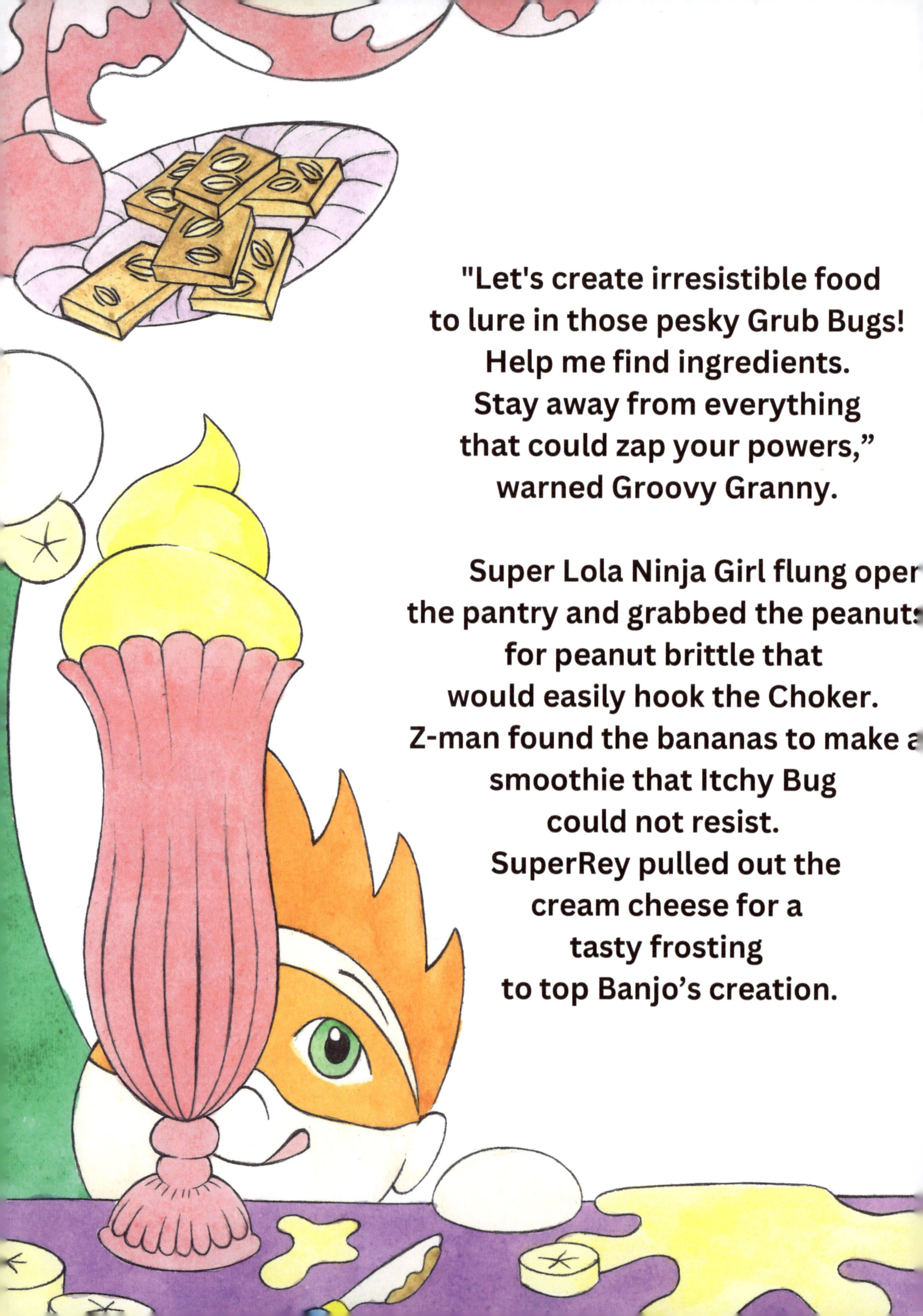

"Let's create irresistible food
to lure in those pesky Grub Bugs!
Help me find ingredients.
Stay away from everything
that could zap your powers,"
warned Groovy Granny.

Super Lola Ninja Girl flung open
the pantry and grabbed the peanuts
for peanut brittle that
would easily hook the Choker.
Z-man found the bananas to make a
smoothie that Itchy Bug
could not resist.
SuperRey pulled out the
cream cheese for a
tasty frosting
to top Banjo's creation.

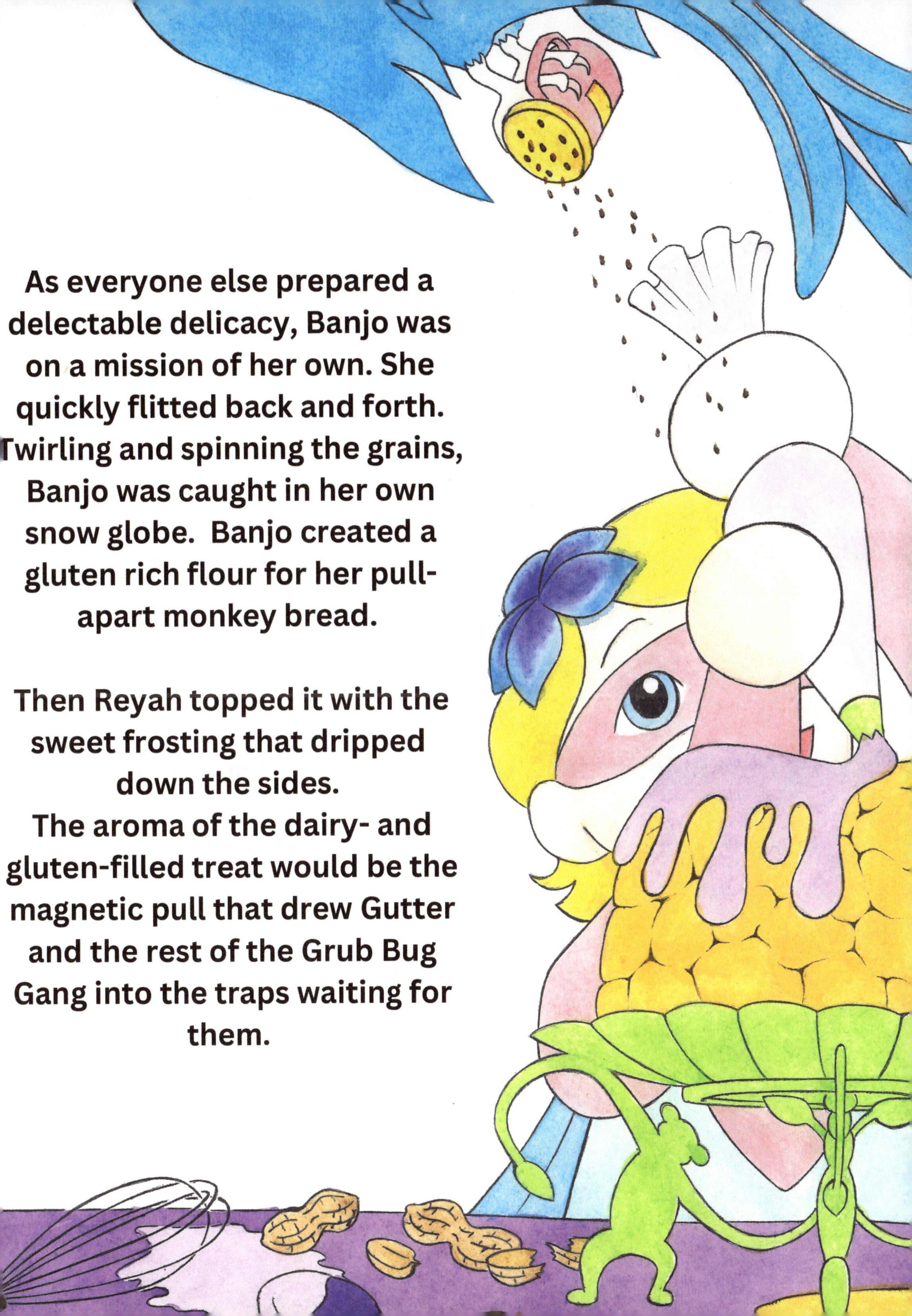

As everyone else prepared a delectable delicacy, Banjo was on a mission of her own. She quickly flitted back and forth. Twirling and spinning the grains, Banjo was caught in her own snow globe. Banjo created a gluten rich flour for her pull-apart monkey bread.

Then Reyah topped it with the sweet frosting that dripped down the sides.
The aroma of the dairy- and gluten-filled treat would be the magnetic pull that drew Gutter and the rest of the Grub Bug Gang into the traps waiting for them.

Suddenly, Banjo fluttered, swirled, and squawked,
**"GROOVY GRANNY! OH NO!
OH NO! GROOOOOVYYYY GRANNNNY!"**

.

Groovy Granny turned and saw El Fuego sneaking across
the yard. It was time!

Groovy Granny snuck over to the freezer and pulled out
the frosty box of ice cream sandwiches. She knew
El Fuego would try to catch her off guard. . .
But not today!

Groovy Granny and the heroes put a stack of ice cream
sandwiches topped with whipped cream on the picnic
table.

Banjo topped them off with a cherry.

Kerplunk!

And then they waited . . .

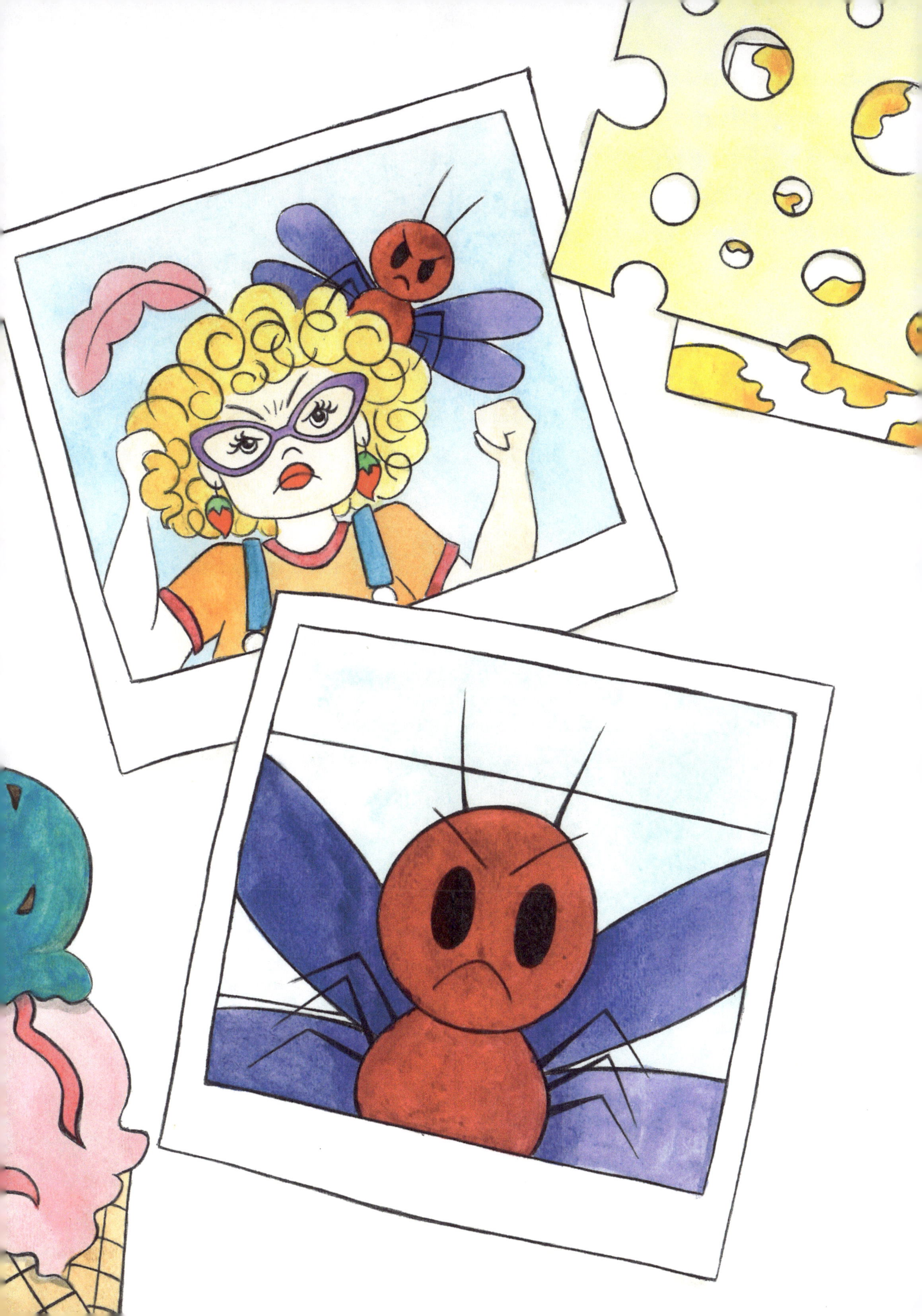

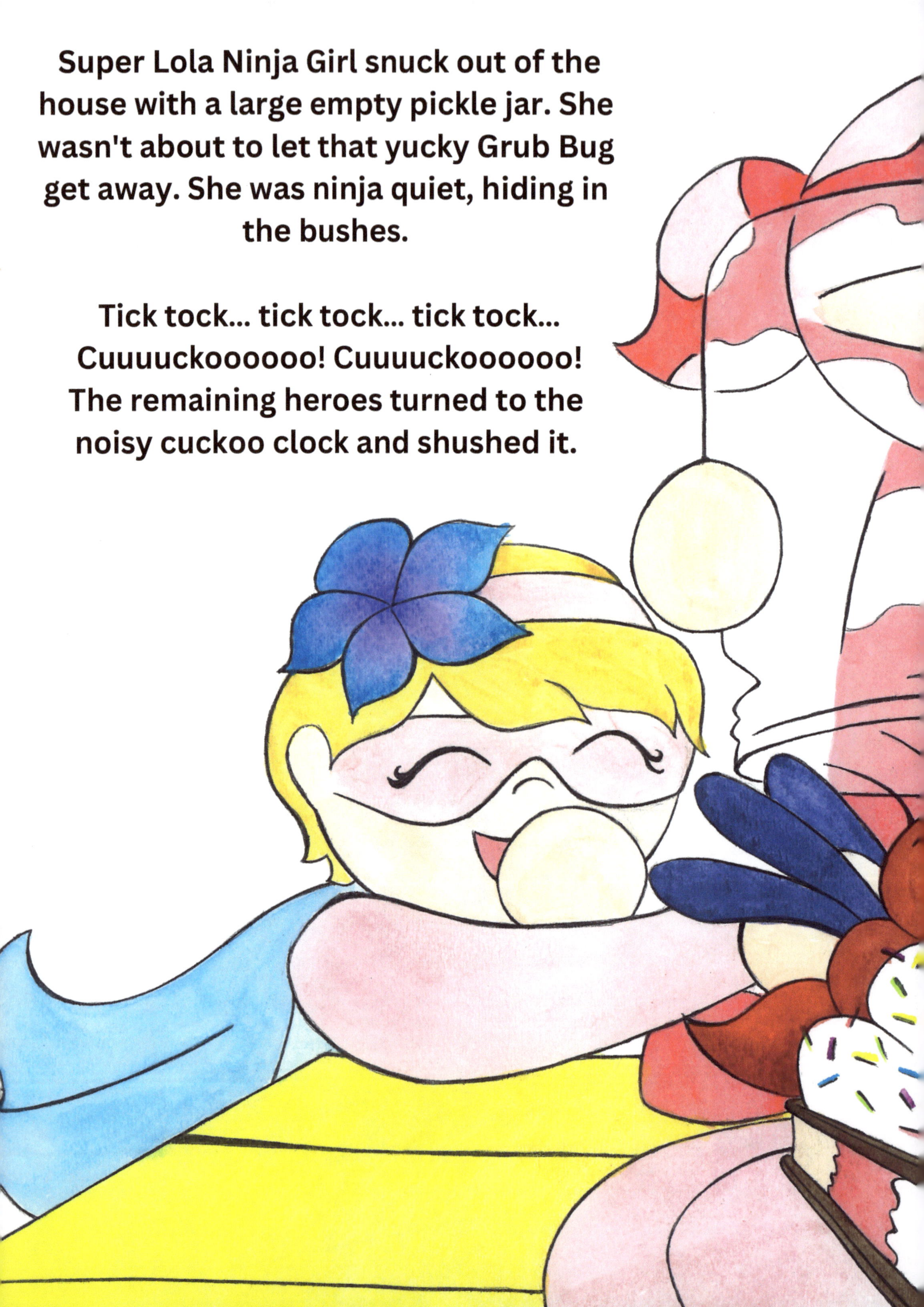

Super Lola Ninja Girl snuck out of the house with a large empty pickle jar. She wasn't about to let that yucky Grub Bug get away. She was ninja quiet, hiding in the bushes.

Tick tock... tick tock... tick tock... Cuuuuckoooooo! Cuuuuckoooooo! The remaining heroes turned to the noisy cuckoo clock and shushed it.

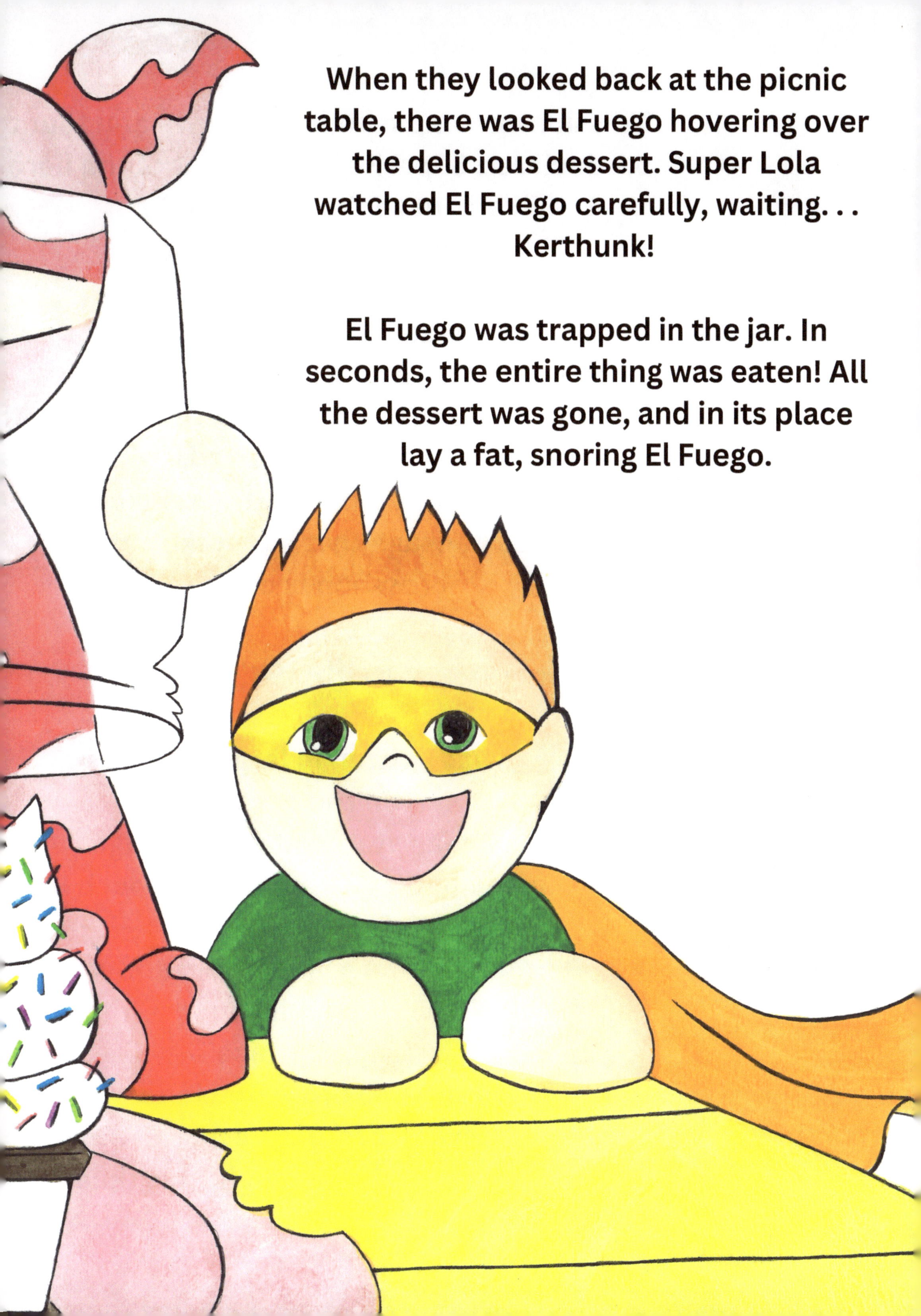

When they looked back at the picnic table, there was El Fuego hovering over the delicious dessert. Super Lola watched El Fuego carefully, waiting. . . Kerthunk!

El Fuego was trapped in the jar. In seconds, the entire thing was eaten! All the dessert was gone, and in its place lay a fat, snoring El Fuego.

"Mission accomplished! One down and four t
go," declared SuperRey as the rest of the hero
ran out to the picnic table.
Super Lola looked worried.

"Oh, don't you worry, sweetie.
It won't be hard at all to catch the rest of
the Grub Bug Gang," comforted Groovy Grann
as she gave her youngest granddaughter a hug
Groovy Granny went to the freezer and too
out a package that had a skull and
crossbones on it.

"POISON!"

was written in large red letters
on the package.
Z-man stared at the package.
He knew what it was and not to touch it!

"Z-man!" came a voice from above.
"Put this on NOW!" Banjo dropped a white clou
on Z-man's face.
This was no ordinary cloud.
It was a protective mask.
He was ready for a fight this time!

Now," said Groovy Granny
"We know El Fuego loved the ice cream sandwich with
whipped cream and a cherry on top
He's safely locked up.
Let's check off the list of Grub Bugs,
making sure we have all the bait to
capture the rest of the gang."

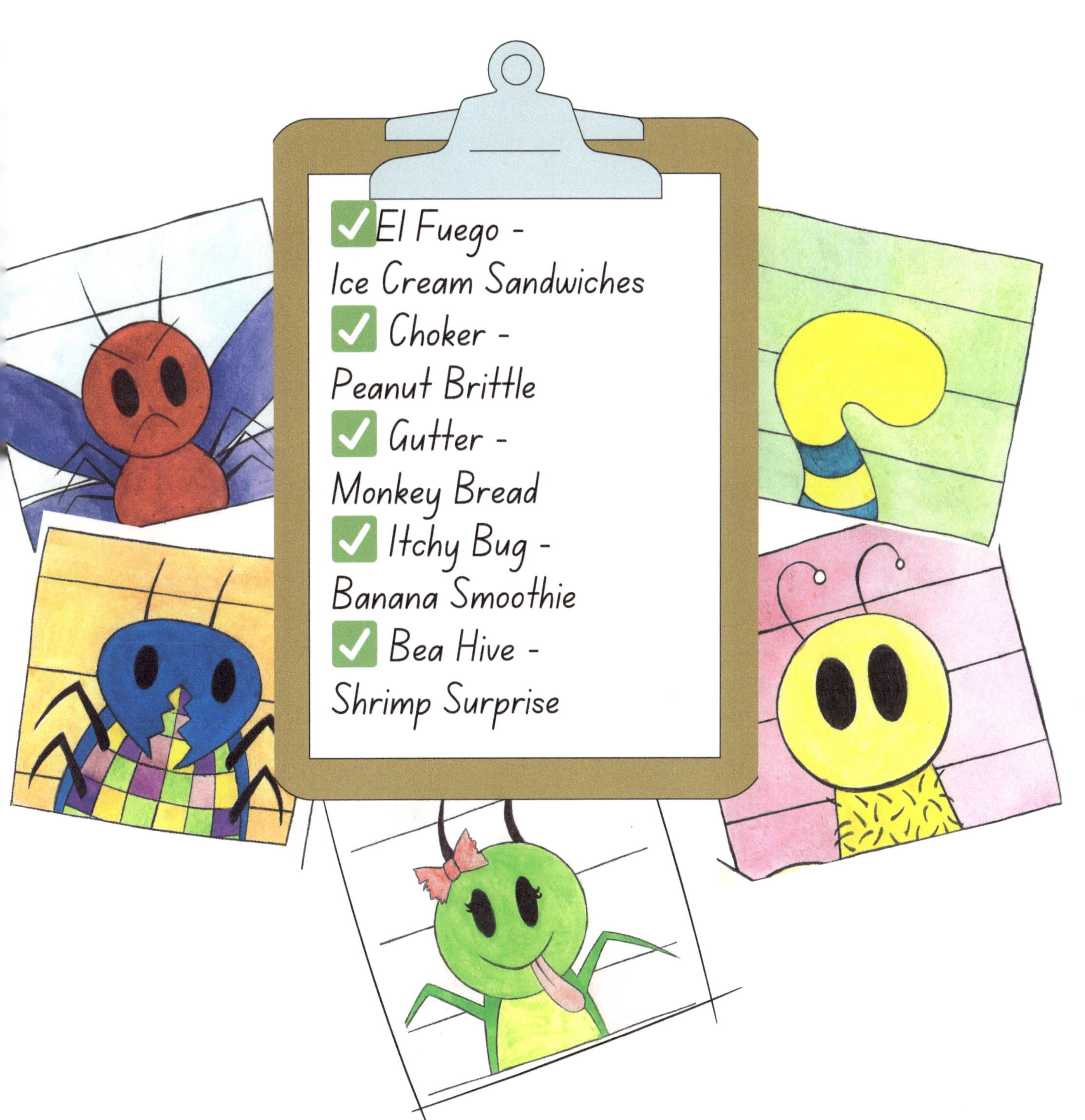

"Ready, my sweet heroes?
Let's hide while the yummy smells do their work,"
Groovy Granny urged, "but be alert
and ready for anything.
This could be quite a battle!"

Banjo was armed with flour bombs to drop on
those Grub Bugs so they couldn't see to escape.
Her eagle eyes scanned the dining room for any
glimpse of those sneaky Grub Bugs.

Lola wielded a rolling pin like a light saber.

Z-man decided to use his speed to
keep the Gang confused.

Groovy Granny opened the tiny prison that would
soon hold the gang that brought
fear and dread everywhere.

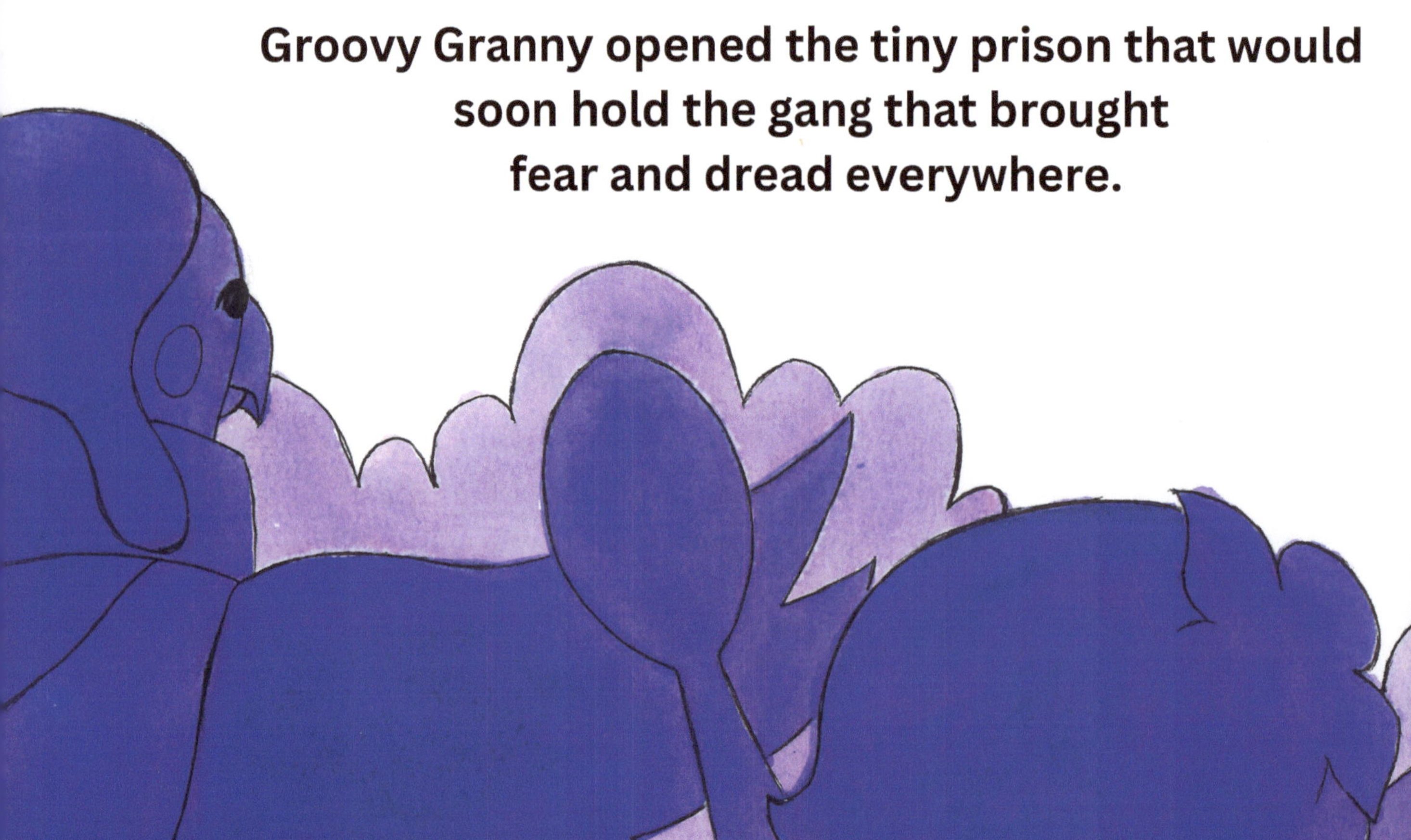

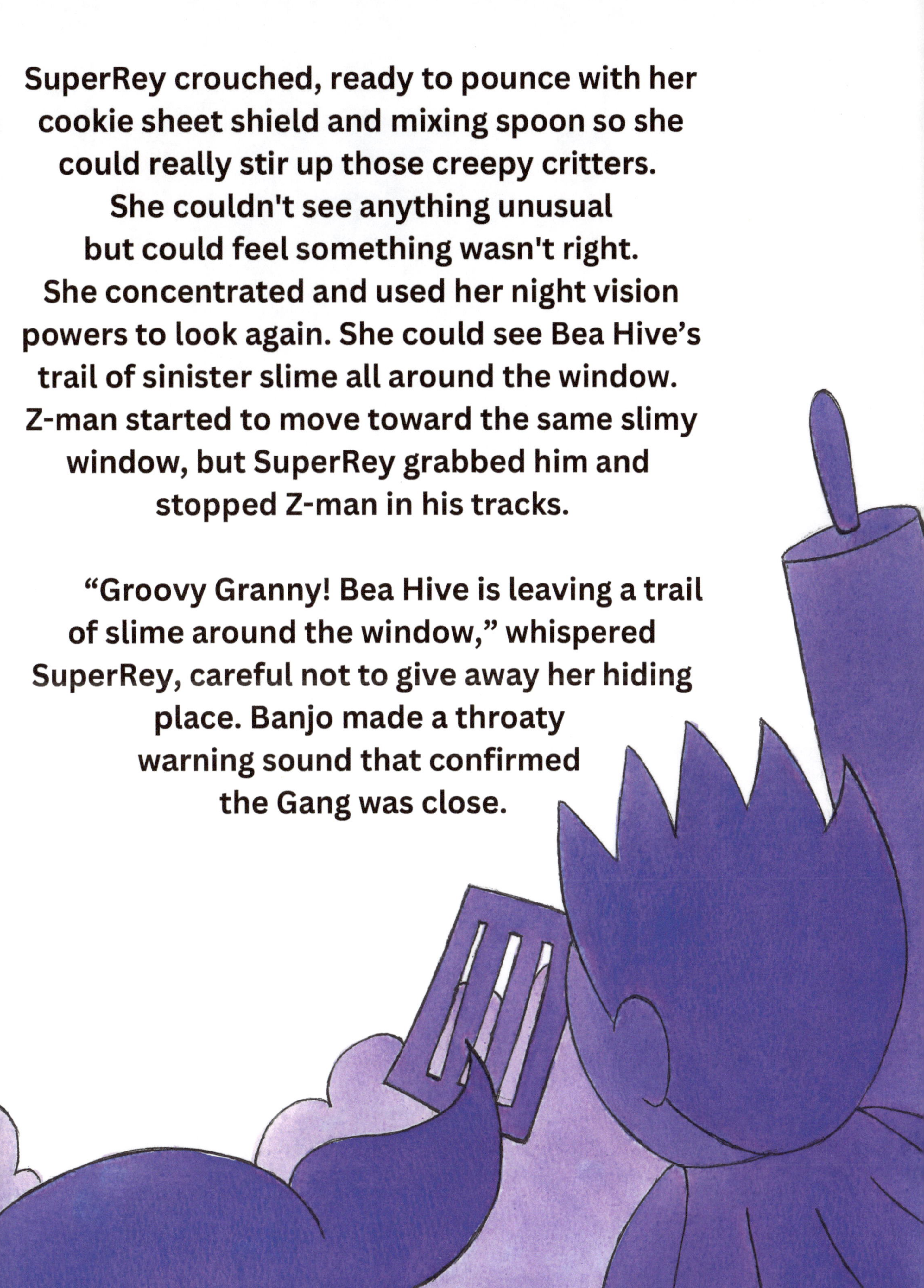

SuperRey crouched, ready to pounce with her cookie sheet shield and mixing spoon so she could really stir up those creepy critters. She couldn't see anything unusual but could feel something wasn't right. She concentrated and used her night vision powers to look again. She could see Bea Hive's trail of sinister slime all around the window. Z-man started to move toward the same slimy window, but SuperRey grabbed him and stopped Z-man in his tracks.

"Groovy Granny! Bea Hive is leaving a trail of slime around the window," whispered SuperRey, careful not to give away her hiding place. Banjo made a throaty warning sound that confirmed the Gang was close.

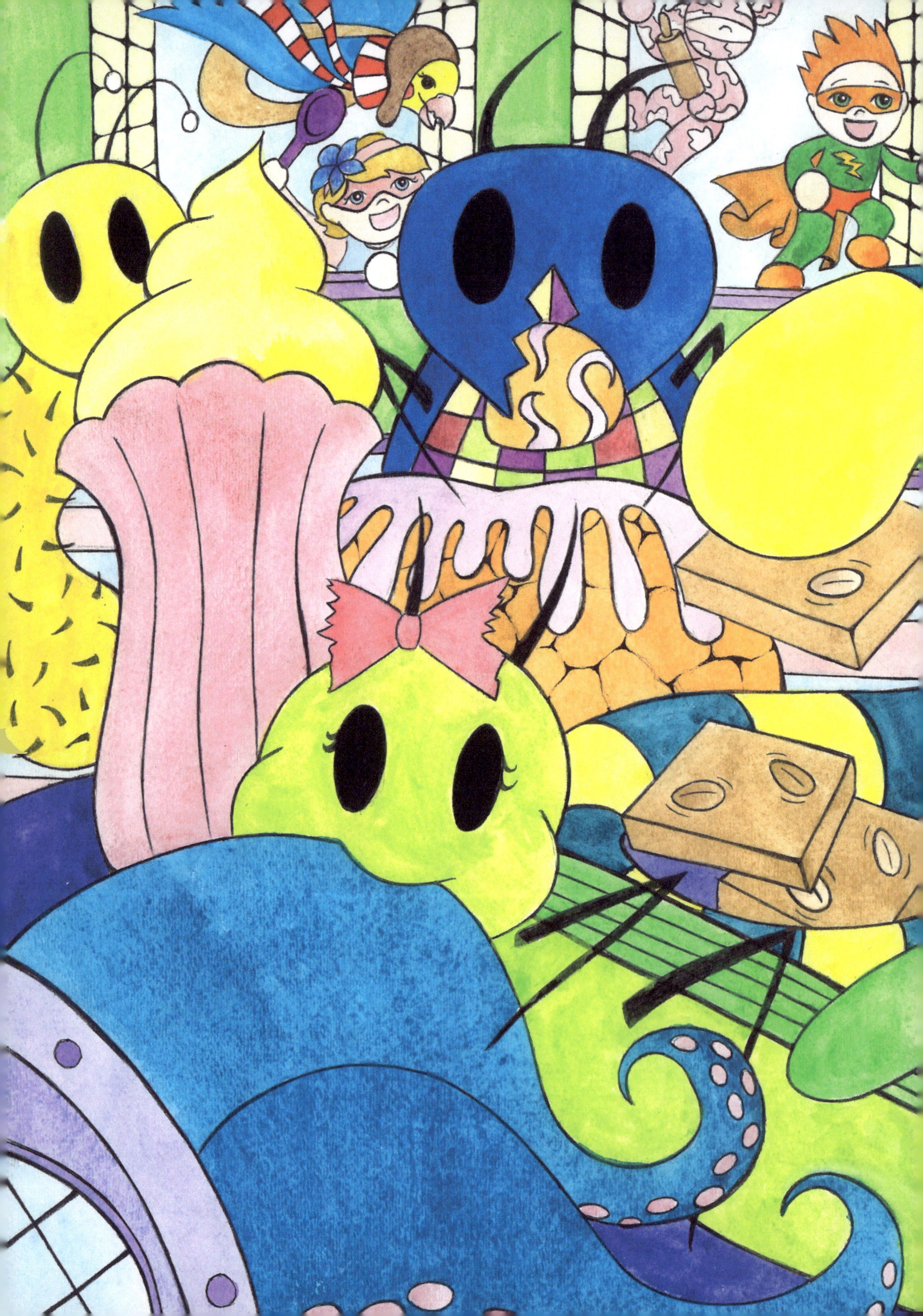

CRRRRUUUUUNNNNNCH!!
Choker had the first bite of the bait!

In one swift swipe, SuperRey scooped up Choker with her mixing spoon, catapulting him right into Super Lola's rolling pin saber.

SCCHHHMACK!

Choker ricocheted off the saber and into the tin box. . . pop went the lid!

"Two down and three to go, my sweet little heroes!" shouted Groovy Granny.

POOOOOWWWWW!!

SuperRey scooped! Ninja Lola schmacked!
Groovy Granny trapped Bea Hive.

"Now, your turn, Gutter! Take that!" Z-man turned the leftover peanut brittle into a catcher's mitt.

THRACK-THRUNK!

Swoosh went SuperRey with the mixing spoon, right to
Ninja Lola. CRAAACK off the rolling pin saber. . .
and SNAP into the trap!

Now it was Itchy Bug's turn. Itchy Bug was swimming
around in the banana smoothie like a
pig in a mudhole.
"Banjo, rodeo up!" Groovy Granny hollered in
her best cowgirl drawl.
Banjo glided in upside down with her scarf held tightly
in her little bird feet, ready to do some fancy ropin'.

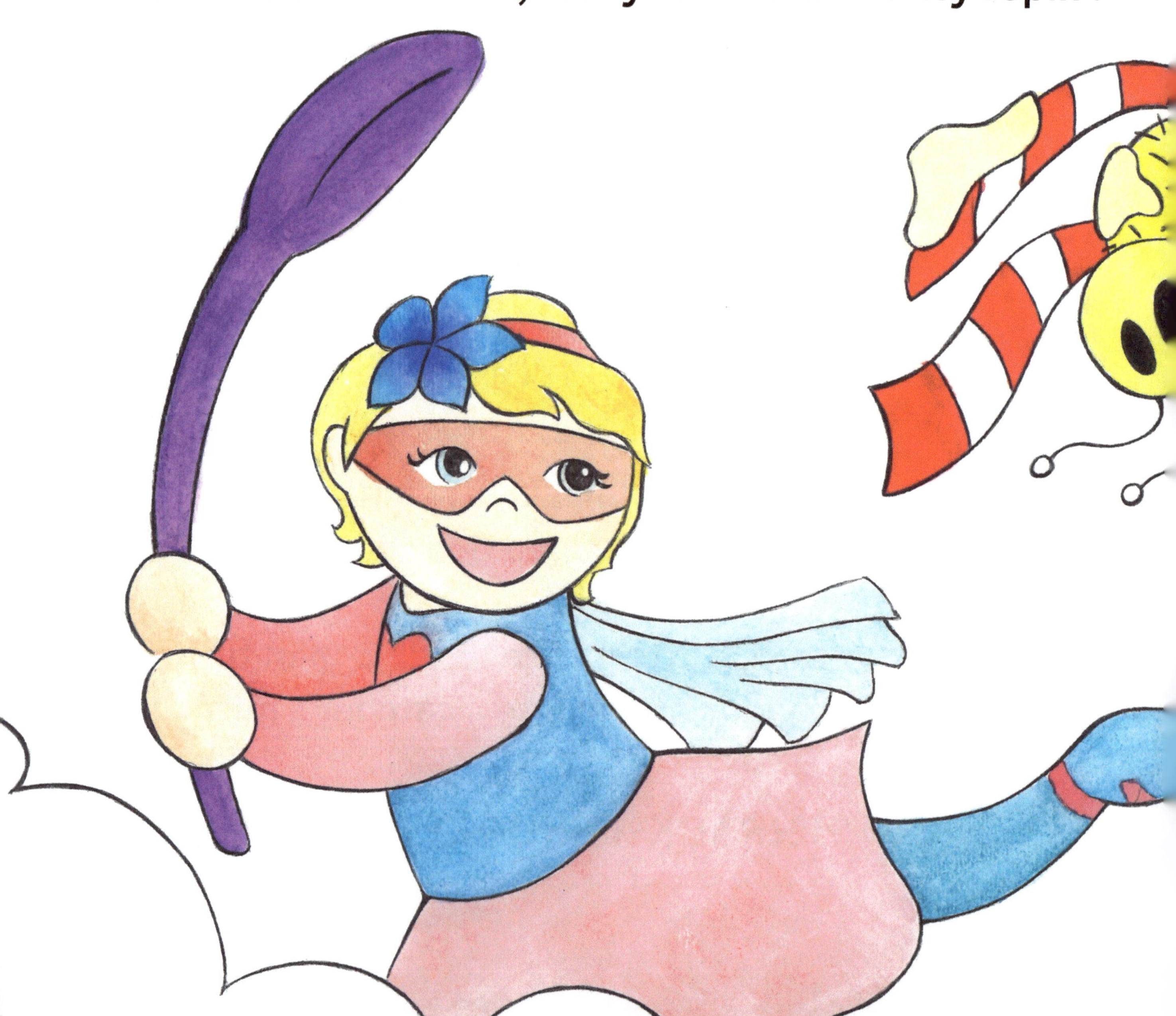

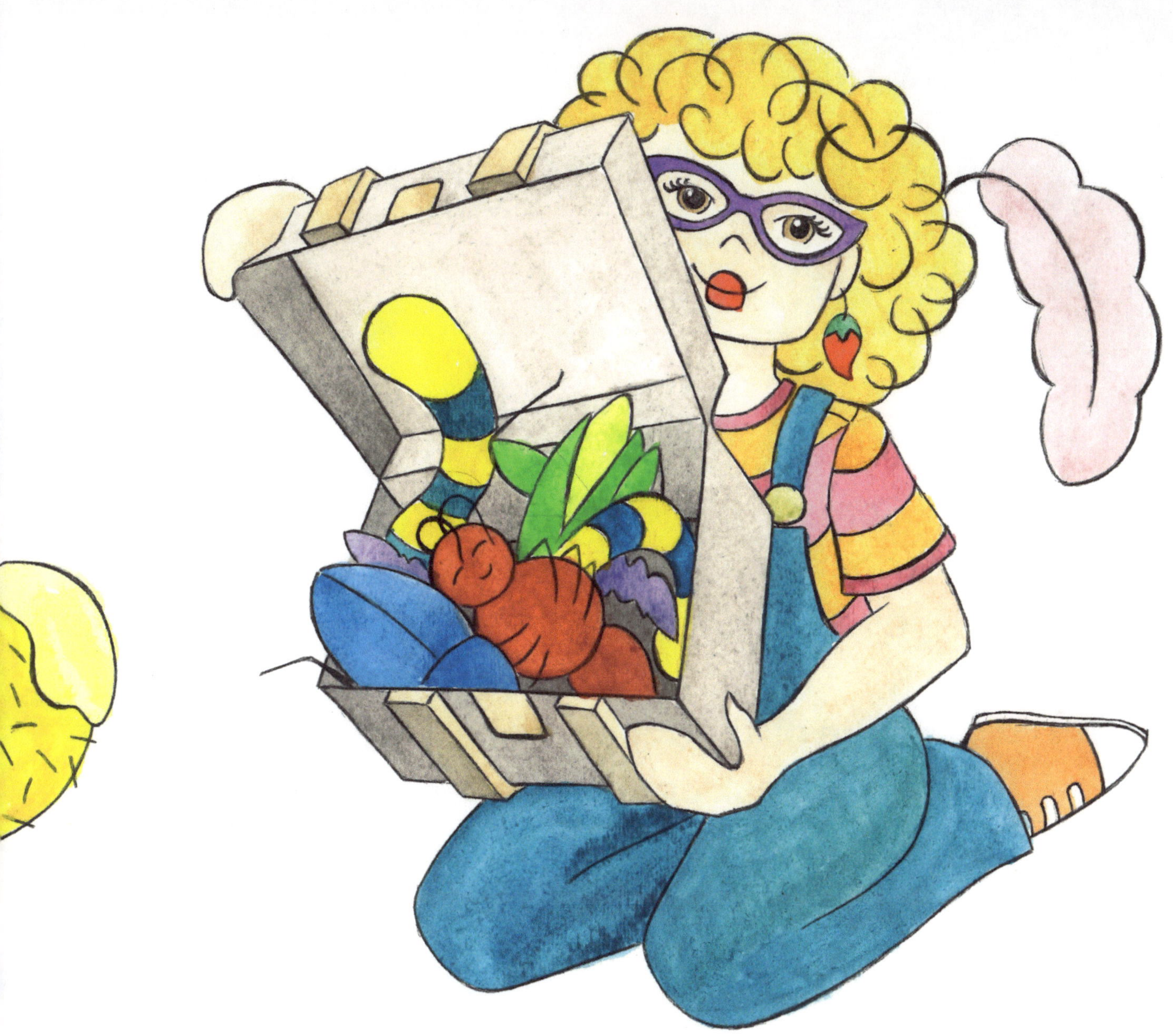

Z-man caught the other end of the scarf as Banjo flew between them, tying Itchy Bug up tight. SuperRey smacked Itchy Bug right into the tin. POP!

"Atta girl, Banjo! 3.8 seconds, and we have the last Grub Bug roped, tied, and pinned!" shouted Z-man. They all whooped and hollered with a yee-haw.

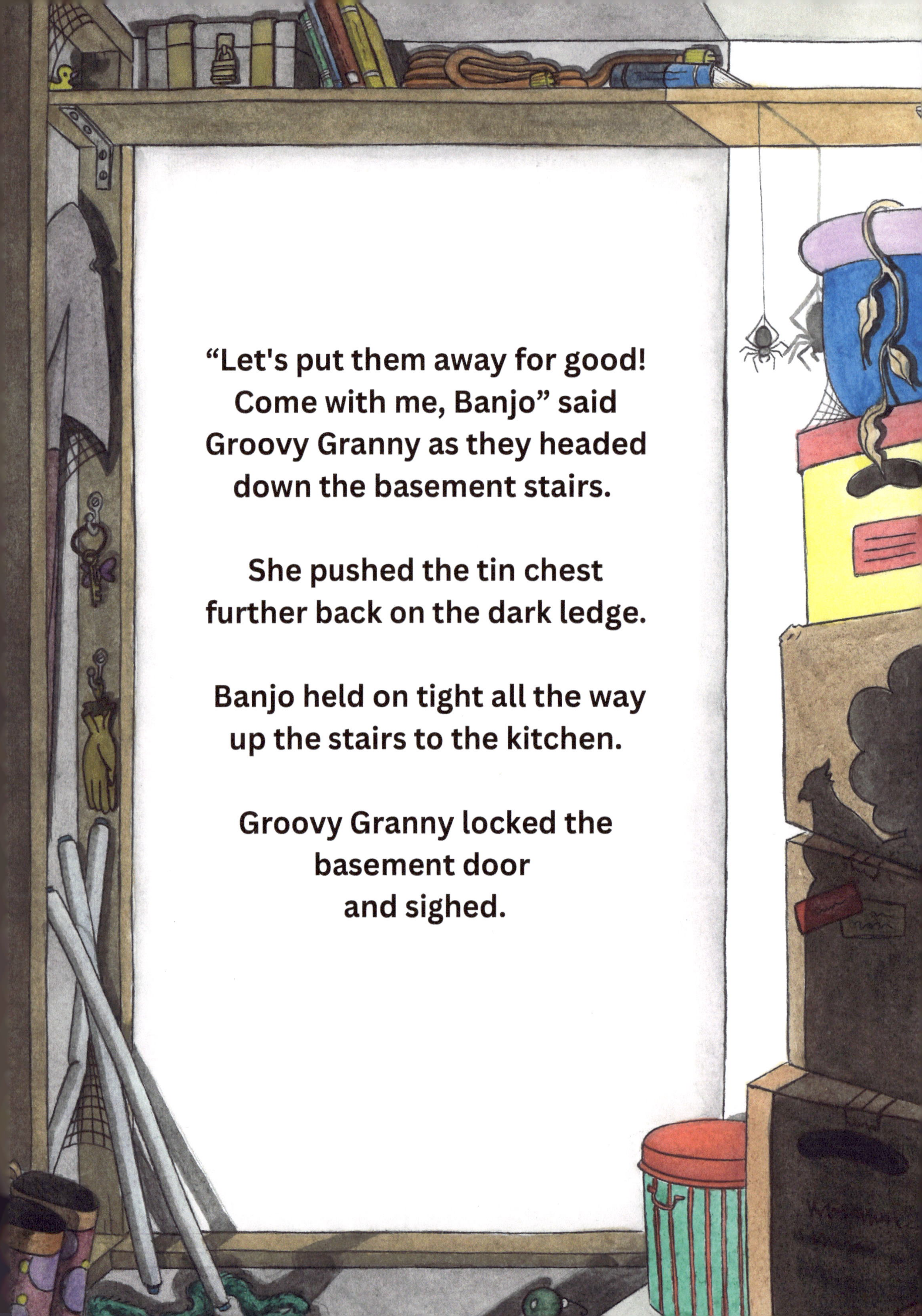

"Let's put them away for good!
Come with me, Banjo" said
Groovy Granny as they headed
down the basement stairs.

She pushed the tin chest
further back on the dark ledge.

Banjo held on tight all the way
up the stairs to the kitchen.

Groovy Granny locked the
basement door
and sighed.

Now it was clean up time.
Everyone worked together to clean the mess.
In a jiffy, it was clean.

With the Grub Bugs locked up
and the party food ready, Lola declared,
"Let's get this party stawted!

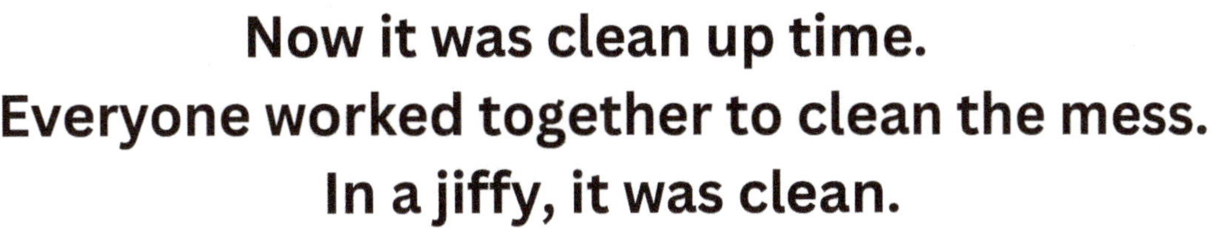

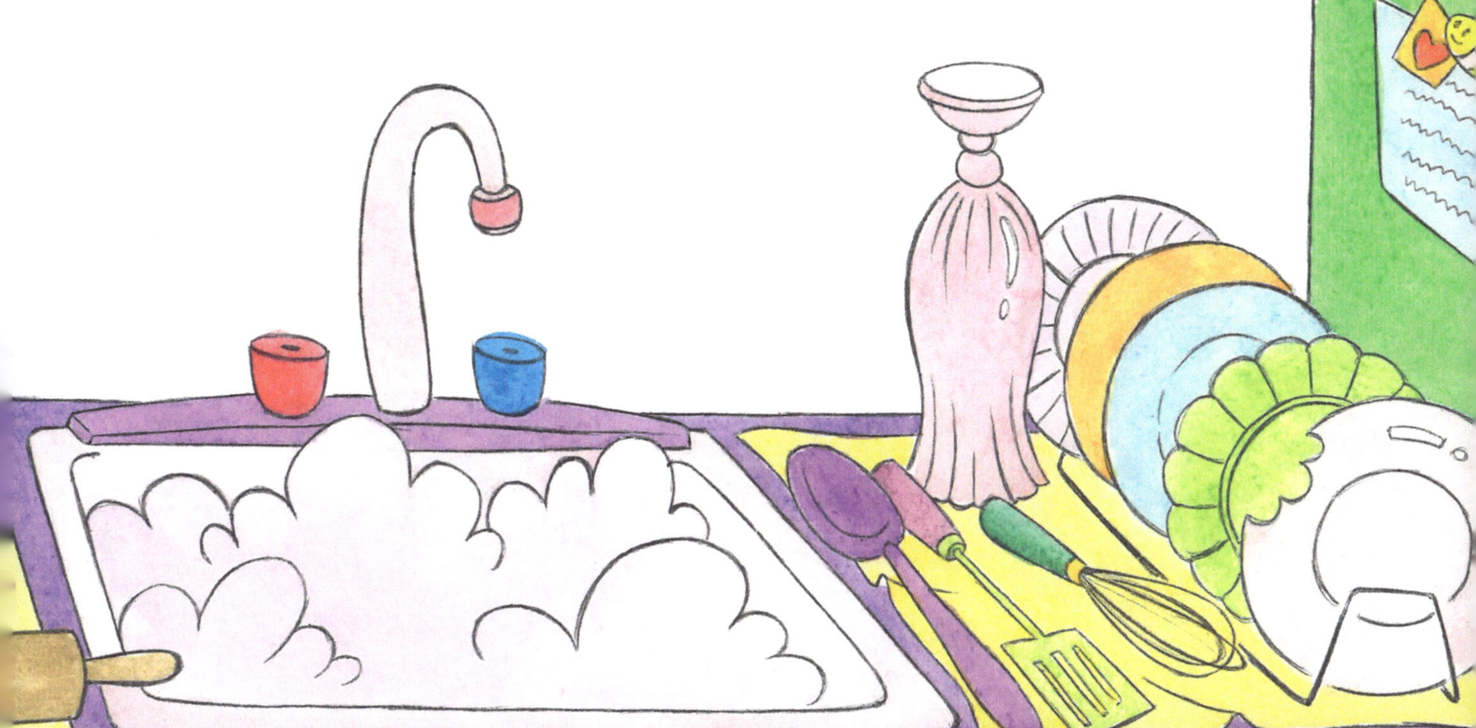

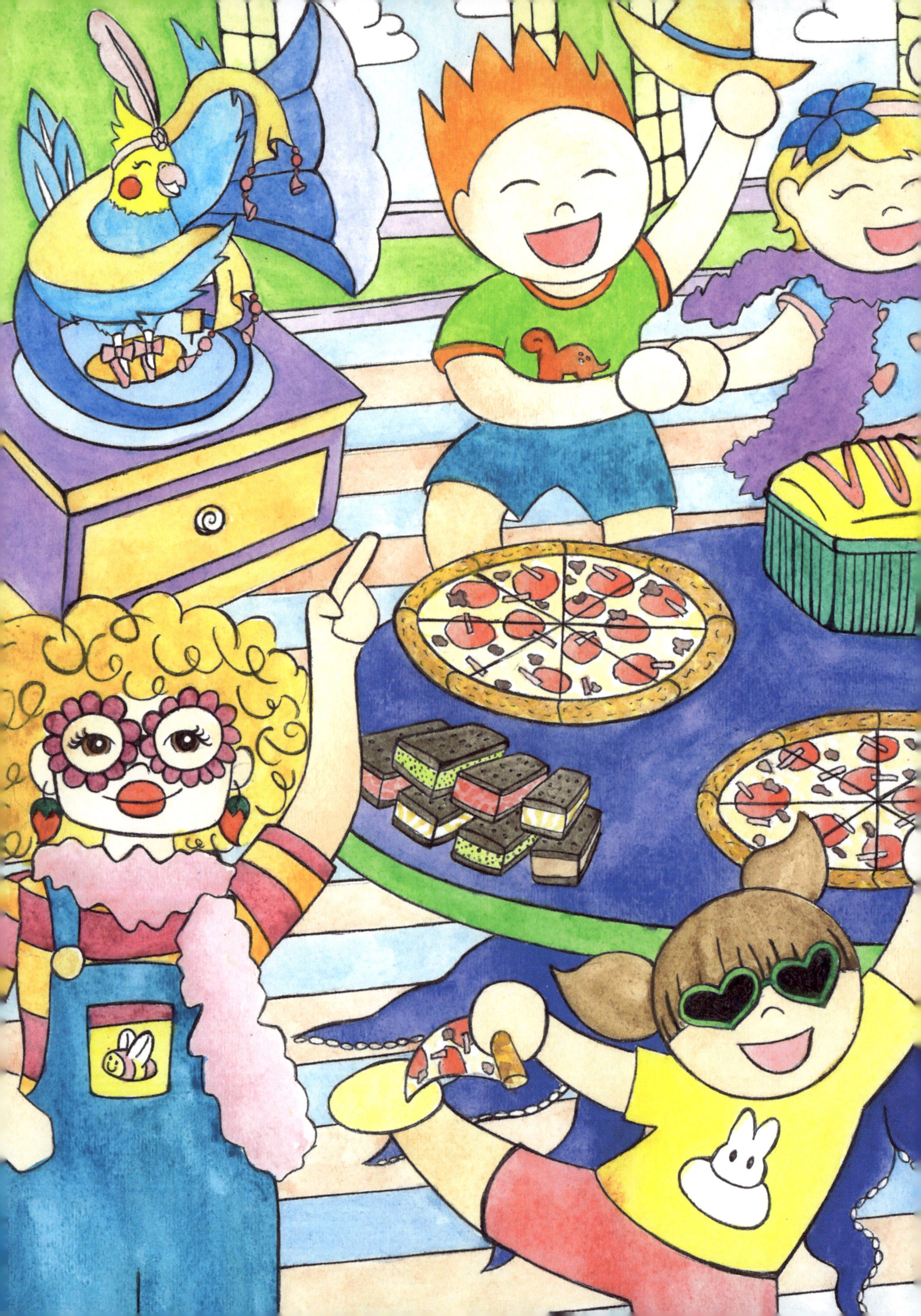

Banjo switched her bomber cap for a tiara.
She was ready to celebrate Banjo-style.
Groovy Granny and Lola brought in the safe foods.

Yummmmm!!

Gluten and lactose free triple meat pizza and the almond milk ice cream sandwiches filled the table.

Banjo turned on the music, and the party began!
She flung open the trunk. She pulled out gratitude glasses, tiaras and cowboy hats for a dance party.

Shake, rattle, and roll!

There was so much happiness going on as everyone danced, sang and laughed, that the whole house shook and rattled from top to bottom!

Little did our Grub Bug fighting heroes know,
down in the basement,
in the darkest corner,
on the top shelf,

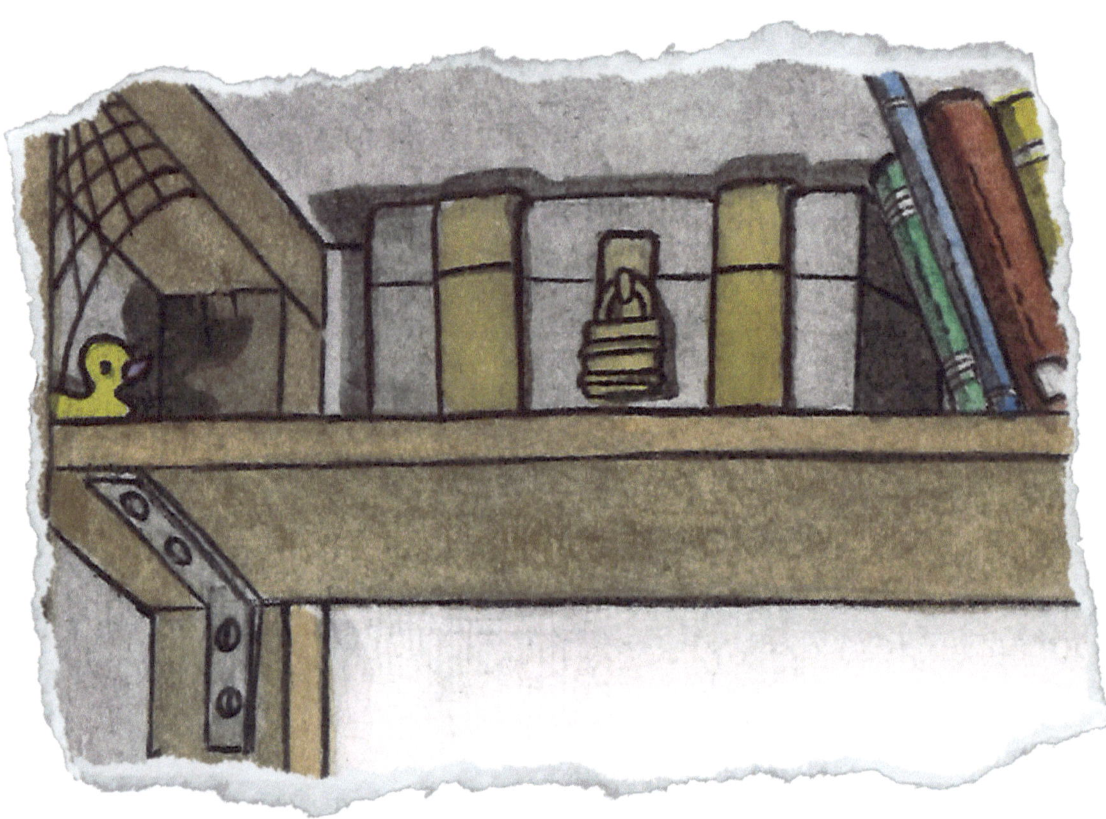

the tin box began to shake. . .

rattle. . .

and roll. . . .

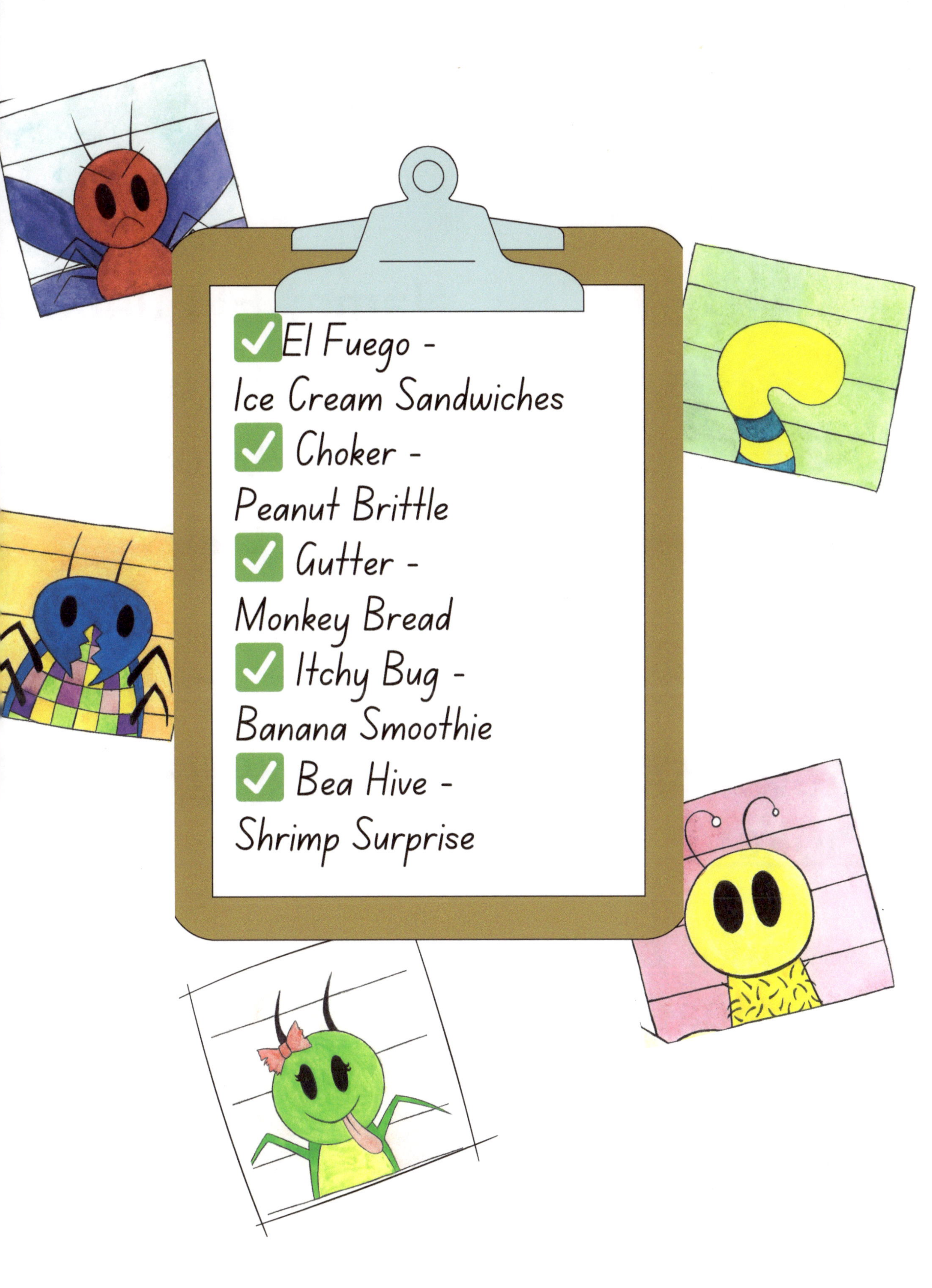

✅El Fuego -
Ice Cream Sandwiches
✅ Choker -
Peanut Brittle
✅ Gutter -
Monkey Bread
✅ Itchy Bug -
Banana Smoothie
✅ Bea Hive -
Shrimp Surprise

Grub Bug Rap Sheet

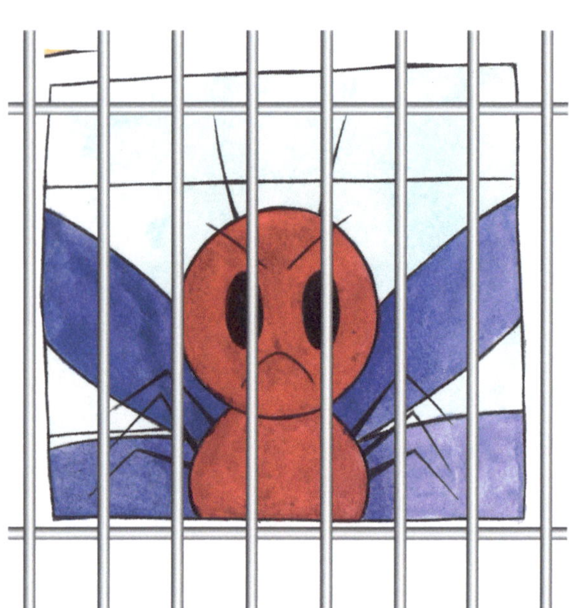

Name: El Fuego
Alias: Firefly
Address: Brown Cow Dairy

Known Associates: <u>Gutter and Choker</u>

Criminal Activity:
- Spreading angry words
- Breaks up friendships
- Favorite food is ice cream sandwiches

Grub Bug Rap Sheet

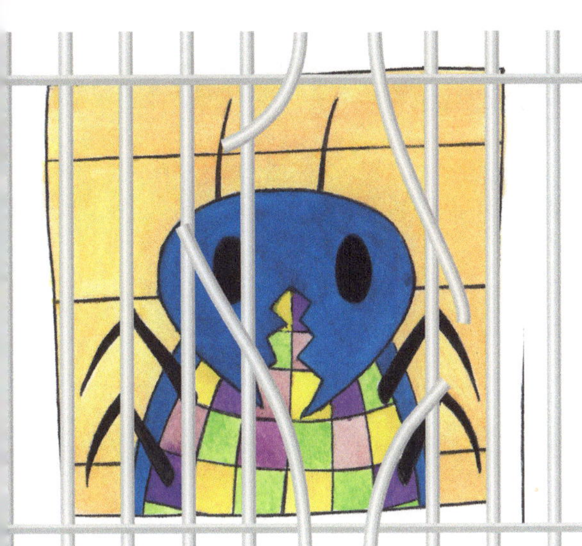

Name: Gutter

Alias: Mr. G

Address: Dough Boy Lane

Known Associates: El Fuego and Choker

Criminal Activity:
- Causes stomachaches
- Causes crankiness
- Favorite food is Monkey Bread

Grub Bug Rap Sheet

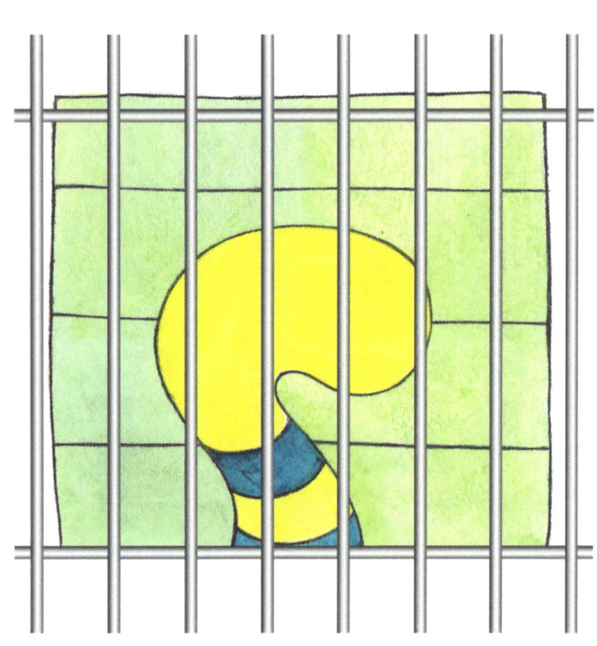

Name: Choker
Alias: Sir Bobble
Address: Peanut Brittle Factory

Known Associates: Choker and Bea Hive

Criminal Activity:
- Scaring little kids
- Pain in the neck
- Favorite food is Peanut Brittle

Grub Bug Rap Sheet

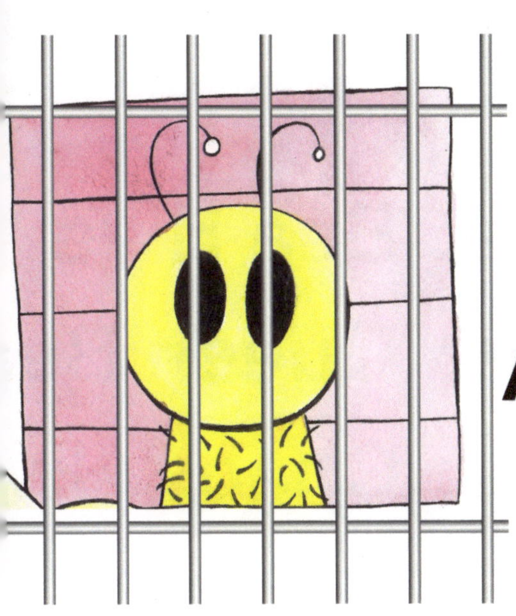

Name: Itchy Bug

Alias: Wiggle Worm

Address: Berkley's Banana Farm

Known Associates: <u>Itchy Bug and Bea Hive</u>

Criminal Activity:

- Causes gurgly and growly sounds
- Causes itchy tongue and throat
- Favorite food is Banana Smoothie

Grub Bug Rap Sheet

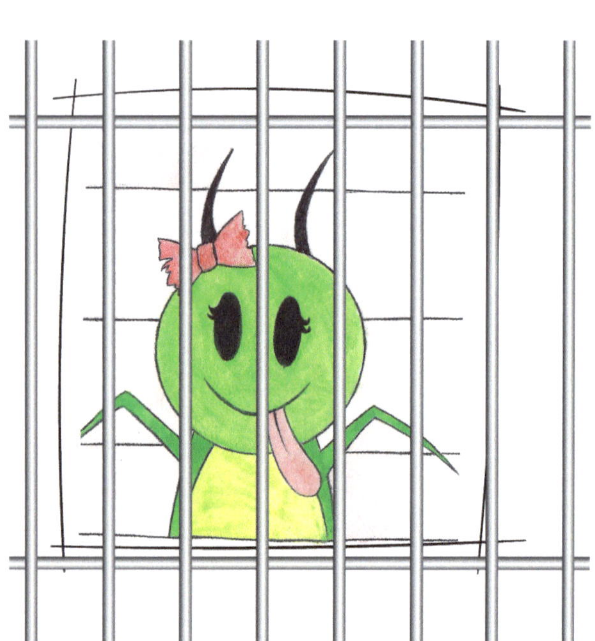

Name: Bea Hive

Alias: Queen Be

Address: Chaos Hiv

Known Associates: <u>Itchy Bug, Gutter and El Fuego</u>

Criminal Activity:
- Causes itchy whelps
- Causes itch and wiggle and wiggle and itch to break out everywhere
- Favorite food is Shrimp Surprise